DR BENJAMIN DANIELS is the pseudonym of a doctor currently working for the NHS.

BENJAMIN DANIELS

Confessions of a GP

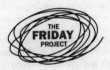

The Friday Project
An imprint of HarperCollins*Publishers*
77–85 Fulham Palace Road
Hammersmith
London W6 8JB

www.harpercollins.co.uk

This edition published by The Friday Project 2012

3

First published in Great Britain by The Friday Project in 2010

A catalogue record for this book is available from the British Library

ISBN 978-1-906321-88-8

Set in Minion 10.5/13.5 pt
Typeset by Palimpsest Book Production Limited, Falkirk, Stirlingshire

Printed and bound in Great Britain by Clays Ltd, St Ives plc

MIX
Paper from
responsible sources
FSC www.fsc.org **FSC® C007454**

Disclaimer

The events described in this book are based on my experiences as a new GP. For obvious reasons of privacy and confidentiality I have made certain changes, altered identifying features and fictionalised some aspects, but it remains an honest reflection of life as a young doctor in Britain today. This is what it's like. These things really happen!

Who am I?

Humans have a universal desire to be listened to and share their stories of pain and suffering. My job as a GP is to listen to those stories. Sometimes I interject with some suggestions or medications, but more often I am simply a passive observer of the soap operas that are people's lives. With regular appointments, I watch the characters develop and the narratives unfold. Although some of my patients have an overinflated view of my significance, I really am just a walk-on part in their lives. I'm like the extra in the corner of the Queen Vic who tries his best to play a small role in one or two of the storylines, but in reality rarely affects the progress of the plot or the big ending. The advantage I do have is that I get to watch the story unfold from a unique and fascinating angle. Being a doctor gives me a privileged insight into the more private and often bizarre aspects of human life and, with that in mind, let me share some slices of my working life with you.

I love my job and have no regrets about choosing to become a doctor and then a GP. This is quite fortunate really, as my decision to study medicine was made as I chose my A levels at the tender age of 16¼. At this time my only real reservation against becoming a doctor was the knowledge that I would have to endure chemistry A level. I couldn't really think of any other reason why I shouldn't be a doctor. What could be better than swanning around a hospital full of beautiful nurses and 'saving lives'? People would think I was great and ultimately this would lead to me finally getting a girlfriend. As an awkward 16-year-old with bad skin and greasy hair, most of my career aspirations were based on what profession would give me the best opportunity of gaining me some interest from the opposite sex. I had accepted that my carnal ambitions would ideally be achieved by being in a boy band or playing Premiership football, but unfortunately my lack of talent in both these departments led to the inevitable choice of medicine. I chose my A levels in the year that *ER* first arrived on our screens. A poster of George Clooney in a white coat was on every girl's wall. Of course I wanted to be a doctor!

On my university application form, I had the good sense to not write that I wanted to be a doctor so I could 'save lives and hence get laid'. I scribbled down something about my love of 'working as part of a team' and my 'fascination with human sciences'. To be fair, I suppose these statements were also true, but it is so hard to pick a career aged 16. The real world of work is always such a mystery until you enter it. When my mate Tom applied to teacher-training college, he wrote that he wanted to 'help young people flourish and fulfil their true potential'. After a five-year tour of duty in an inner city comprehensive school, like us medics, he is just trying to get to the weekend without being punched or sued.

Although I'm now a GP, my training required me to spend many long years working as a hospital doctor. I completed five years at medical school and then spent several years working in various hospital posts gaining the experience needed to become a GP. I was a junior doctor in surgery, psychiatry, A&E, paediatrics, gynaecology, geriatrics and general medicine. I also broke up my training with a three-month stint working in Mozambique. All in all I loved working as a hospital doctor but have absolutely no regrets about leaving it to become a GP.

Introduction

I can still fondly recall the first diagnosis I ever made. As with many others that followed, it was spectacularly incorrect, but it still holds a special place in my heart. In my defence, I was just a mere boy at the time, wet behind the ears and only a few weeks into my first term at medical school. I was sitting in the local Kentucky Fried Chicken and spotted a man slumped unconscious in his plastic seat. A wave of excitement flooded over me. This was what it was all about! This was my vocation! With the limitless enthusiasm of youth and inexperience, I bounded over to undoubtedly save his life with my new-found wealth of medical knowledge.

It didn't take me long to conclude that this gent had suffered from a spontaneous pneumothorax. This was not based on clinical signs and symptoms but more that this was the condition that we had learnt about that morning in a tutorial and so was the first and only diagnosis that sprung to mind. With an air of self-importance, I explained to the KFC manager my diagnosis and instructed him to call urgently for an ambulance. Looking thoroughly unimpressed, he wandered out from behind the counter and roughly manhandled the unconscious man from his seat and threw him out of his restaurant. My first-ever patient spectacularly regained consciousness, uttered a few obscenities addressed to no one in particular and staggered off down the street. The KFC manager in his far superior wisdom had, in fact, made the correct diagnosis of 'drunk and asleep' and prescribed him a swift exit from his premises.

I can see why the professor chose to teach us innocent medical students about a spontaneous pneumothorax that morning. It is, in fact, a wonderful feel-good condition for doctors. An otherwise healthy person collapses with a deflated lung and then the clever doctor diagnoses it with his stethoscope and sticks a needle between their ribs. With a triumphant hissing sound, the lung inflates and the patient feels much better. The professor was trying to help explain the normal functioning of the lung and what could go wrong. He was also trying to encourage us to embrace the wonderful healing abilities we could have as doctors. Back during those early days of medical school I believed that most of medicine would be that straightforward. Someone would be unwell, I would do something fabulous and then they would get better.

Funnily enough, despite a spontaneous pneumothorax being the first medical condition I ever learnt about at medical school, I have, in fact, never actually seen one since. Looking back, I wonder if actually a far more useful and accurate introduction to being a front line NHS doctor would have been a tutorial on how to remove a semiconscious drunk bloke from a waiting room:

'Would everyone please welcome our guest speaker today. He has a long and celebrated career working in numerous late-night fast food outlets and will be giving you his annual demonstration on how to prepare yourselves for spending your futures working in the NHS. Do take notes on how he skilfully removes the inebriated gentleman while remaining entirely unsoiled by any body fluids and simultaneously evading drunken punches. You will be tested on this in your end-of-year exams, so do pay attention.'

When I think back to that KFC, I can still recall my shock at what I perceived to be the terrible ill treatment of this poor man.

The callous, heartless actions of the restaurant manager only increased the feeling that my true vocation was to become an amazing doctor in order to cure just such vulnerable people who needed my help . . .

Ten years later, after a long day of inner city general practice, my brain was heavy with the multitude of sufferings that I had encountered. Chronic pains, domestic violence, addiction, depression, self-harming and a fairly big helping of broad-spectrum misery were the principal orders of the day. After many hours of putting my heart and soul into my patients' problems, I knew that my competency that day would be judged not on my diagnostic skills or my bedside manner, but by how many targets I had reached from the latest pointless government directive. While finishing the day reading the latest newspaper headline about how GPs were lazy money-grabbers, it was almost a relief to receive an emergency call from reception to tell me that a man had collapsed in the waiting room.

Rather than springing up into life-saving action, I heaved myself out of my blissfully comfortable chair and ambled down to the waiting room. Over the last ten years that limitless enthusiasm had been gradually broken down and replaced with a defeated resignation. I took no satisfaction in this time getting my diagnosis spot on. Still waiting for that spontaneous pneumothorax to heroically cure, I was greeted instead by one of our local street drinkers in a drunken stupor in the children's play area of the waiting room. Using the expertise I perfected during endless Friday and Saturday night shifts in A&E, I skilfully escorted the intoxicated man from the surgery back on to the street.

In a wave of sad nostalgia I wondered what that naïve 18-year-old me would think about what he had become. Would I have even bothered to have gone on to study medicine if I could have foreseen how so much of that initial hope and optimism would drain away? Not even out of my twenties yet, I began to wonder if being a doctor was anything close to the career I thought it was going to be. As I returned the drunk homeless man on to the street, I offered him an appointment to come back and see me the following morning when he was sober, explaining about organising an alcohol detox. 'I'll be there, Doc,' he told me as he shoved the appointment card into his pocket. We both knew that he'd miss that appointment, but at least we were mutually left with a faint glimmer of hope for something better.

Please don't imagine that this book is about me looking for sympathy or commiserations about my broken dreams, or assume that I have lost my empathy and respect for the people who expectantly seek my help or advice. I guess it's just that the often grim reality of practising inner city medicine is not quite what I had expected it to be. I no longer dream of miracle cures and magic bullets and I have definitely given up waiting to dramatically re-inflate that collapsed lung. Instead, I acknowledge that my role is to listen and share the pains, concerns and sufferings of the people who sit before me. I offer the odd nugget of good advice and provide some support at times of need. Perhaps just occasionally I even make a small difference in someone's life. The intention of this book is simply to give an honest but light-hearted insight into some of the joys, frustrations and absurdities of being an inner city NHS GP today. I hope you enjoy it.

I have only been a GP for three years but I do genuinely love the job. I like the variety and getting to know my patients. I find it challenging and rewarding. Sometimes I even make a diagnosis and cure someone! I'm currently working as a locum which means that I work in different GP surgeries in different parts of the country, covering other GPs when they are away. I also still do some shifts as an A&E doctor from time to time. Some of my posts have just been for one day, others have been for over a year and I get to see the good, bad and ugly side of general practice, patients and the NHS. I love my job and think that it is one of the most interesting out there. I hope that after reading this book you might agree with me, or if not at least realise that it isn't just about seeing coughs and colds.

Mrs Peacock

Like parents, doctors are not supposed to have favourites but I have to admit to being rather fond of Mrs Peacock. She is well into her eighties and her memory has been deteriorating over the last few years. Most weeks she develops a medical problem and calls up the surgery requesting me to visit. When I arrive, the medical problem has been resolved or at least forgotten and I end up changing the fuse on the washing machine or helping her to find her address book, which we eventually locate in the fridge. As I tuck into a milky cup of tea and a stale coconut macaroon, I reflect that my medical skills probably aren't being put to best use. I imagine the grumbling taxpayer wouldn't be too pleased to know that having forked out over £250,000 to put me through my medical school training, they are now paying my high GP wages in order for me to ineptly try to recall which coloured wire is earth in Mrs Peacock's ageing plug.

Mrs Peacock needs a bit of social support much more than she needs a doctor so when I return to the surgery I spend 30 minutes trying to get through to social services on the phone. When I finally get through, I am told that because of her dementia, Mrs Peacock needs a psychiatric assessment before they can offer any social assistance. The psychiatrist is off sick with depression and the waiting list to see the stand-in psychiatrist is three months. I'm also reminded that Mrs Peacock will need to have had a long list of expensive tests to exclude a medical cause for her memory loss. Three months and many normal test results later, Mrs Peacock forgot to go to her appointment and had to return to the back of the queue.

Through no fault of her own, Mrs Peacock has cost the NHS a small fortune. Her heart scan, blood tests and hospital appointments all cost money and we GPs don't come cheap, either. Mrs Peacock does have mild dementia but more importantly she is lonely. She needs someone to pop in for a cup of tea from time to time and remind her to feed her long-suffering cat. It would appear that this service is not on offer, so, in the meantime, I'll continue to visit from time to time. When the coconut macaroons become so inedible that even the hungry cat won't eat them, I'll think again about trying to get Mrs Peacock some more help.

Tom Jones

The term 'presenting complaint' is what we use when we describe what the patient comes in complaining about – i.e. the patient's words rather than our diagnosis. Normally as a GP the presenting complaint will be 'back pain' or 'earache' or 'not sleeping'. Elaine Tibb's presenting complaint was different. When I said, 'Hello Miss Tibbs. What can I help you with today?' she said, 'I'm having pornographic dreams about Tom Jones.' Her words, not mine.

For the more common presenting complaints, most doctors will already have a check list of questions in their heads. For example, a female patient says, 'I've got tummy pain' and I say, 'Where, and for how long?' and 'Have you got any vaginal discharge?' When faced with the presenting complaint of pornographic dreams about a celebrity, I was left hopelessly speechless. When discussing Elaine's sexual fantasies, I was very keen not to know where, for how long and if there had been any vaginal discharge. Unfortunately, I didn't get a chance to point this out to Elaine before every minuscule aspect of the dreams was described in surprisingly graphic detail.

I am rarely left speechless by a patient's opening gambit, but as with Elaine, there are always a few that do leave me at a complete loss. My personal favourites are:

When I eat a lot of rice cakes, it makes my wee smell of rice cakes;

I masturbate 10 to 15 times per day – what should I do?

I ate four Easter eggs this morning and now I feel sick;

My husband can't satisfy me sexually;

When I was in church this morning, I was overcome by the power of the Lord;

I think my vagina is haunted.

Elaine is a classic example of someone that we GPs see fairly regularly. She was odd and eccentric, but not quite mentally ill. She was slightly obsessive and delusional but not really harming herself or anyone else. Admittedly she didn't work, but she functioned reasonably well from day to day and didn't really have any insight into the fact that other people found her to be a tad unusual. Instead, Elaine generally saw most of the rest of the world as slightly peculiar and felt it was just her and, of course, her darling Tom Jones who were the only normal ones. Looking through her patient records, I noted that she did once see a psychiatrist a few years back. He diagnosed her as having 'some abnormal and obsessive personality traits but no active psychosis'. This is psychiatry speak for 'slightly odd but basically harmless'

'He does love me, you know, Doctor. If he met me, he would know it straight away. We're made for each other.'

'Isn't Tom Jones happily married and living in America?'

'No no no! He loves me, doctor.' Elaine would have happily spent all afternoon telling me about her Tom Jones fantasies, but I felt that we needed to move things on. I used the classic GP phrase that we pull out of the bag when we feel that we're not getting very far. 'So Elaine, what are you hoping that I'm going to do for you today?'

'Well, doctor, I need you to write Tom a letter. It would sound better coming from you. He's a doctor as well. Well, not a real doctor, but I'm sure he'd be a wonderful doctor if he wanted to be. He's very kind you know and oooh so gorgeous and anyway, I'm sure if you just explained everything he would see sense, I know he would.'

Basically, I was being asked to stalk Tom Jones on Elaine's behalf. I could imagine the letter.

Dear Tom,
Please will you leave your wife, family and LA mansion and move into a council bedsit with a slightly odd woman with straggly hair and a duffel coat that she has been wearing since 1983. It will make my life slightly easier as she won't keep coming to the surgery and annoying me with her graphic descriptions of your imaginary sex life.
  Best wishes,
  Dr Daniels

Stalking is defined as a 'constellation of behaviours in which an individual inflicts upon another repeated unwanted intrusions and communications'. Elaine probably would have quite liked to have stalked Tom Jones, but I don't think she really had it in her. For Elaine, her problems with relating to everyday folk had resulted in her focusing all her energy on an imaginary relationship with a person whom she would never meet. I guess this was a good way to protect herself from the struggles and potential rejections of real-life relationships. Whatever the psychological explanation, I'll never be able to listen to 'It's Not Unusual' in quite the same way again.

Targets

Lucy, the practice manager, popped her head around the door: 'I've put you down for a visit to see Mrs Tucker. She's had a funny turn and fallen over. Perhaps you could diagnose her as having had a stroke?'

It is January and our Quality and Outcomes Framework (QOF) targets are due in April. None of our patients has had a stroke in the last nine months. This should, of course, be a cause for celebration, but Lucy is not happy. If no one has a stroke before April, we will miss out on our 'stroke target'. The government tells us that if a patient has a stroke, we need to refer him/her to the stroke specialist and then we'll get five points! But if no one has a stroke, we miss out on the points and the money that comes with them. The more QOF points the practice earns, the more money the partners take home as profit. The practice manager also takes her cut as an Easter bonus if the surgery gets maximum points. In the world of general practice, points really do mean prizes.

Some older GPs hate disease guidelines. They feel that they take away our autonomy as doctors and rob us of our integrity and ability to make our own clinical decisions. I myself don't begrudge guidelines at all. Strokes have been poorly managed in the community for years and some good research has shown that if someone has a stroke or a mini stroke and we sort out their cholesterol and blood pressure and send them to see a stroke specialist, we can genuinely reduce the chance of them having another stroke.

Mrs Tucker is 96 and lives in a nursing home nearby. She is severely demented and doesn't know her own name. In her confusion she wanders around the nursing home and frequently takes a tumble. She had fallen over again today and could well have had a mini stroke. Having said that, she could just as easily have simply tripped over a stray Zimmer frame or slipped on a rogue Murray Mint. She was back to her normal self now and common sense told me that this lady would not benefit from a whole load of tests and new medications that in the long run would probably only increase her confusion and make her more likely to fall over.

I'm allowed to be puritanical because I'm not a partner and so don't make any money from the QOF points. But would I have been tempted to diagnose Mrs Tucker as having had a stroke if I knew it meant that I would pocket some extra cash in April? Amazingly, in the vast majority of practices that I have worked in, the doctors are incredibly honest about achieving their targets truthfully. However, shouldn't we remove the temptation altogether? Surely, doctors should be able to make sensible decisions about what is in the best interest of our patients without needing targets and cash incentives?

First day

I can still remember my first day as a doctor very clearly. It is something that I had been looking forward to since I first chose my A level subjects eight years earlier. Now the actual day had finally come I was absolutely shitting myself and wondering if I wanted to be there at all. We spent most of the first day having induction-type talks. These consisted of a fire safety talk and an introduction from a medical lawyer on how best not to get sued. Not particularly confidence boosting.

As the induction day drew to a close, most of the other new doctors went to the pub. Not me though. I was doing my first 'on call' on my first-ever night as a doctor. This may have been the short straw for some but, although frightened, I was excited and keen to get my first on call over with. This night would be the making of me, I thought to myself. By this time tomorrow, I would be feeling like an old pro and be regaling heroic stories of my life-saving antics to my admiring colleagues in the pub. It was going to be like losing my virginity all over again. My brand-new shirt was ironed and although a couple of sizes too big, my white coat was starched and gleaming. I had a sensible haircut and a stethoscope round my neck. I looked at myself in the mirror astounded that I really was a doctor!

21

I picked up my pager at five that evening and sat there looking at it timidly. This small black box would come to be hated by me during my future years as a hospital doctor. This box would wake me from sleep and interrupt my meals. When completely overloaded with work and feeling like I couldn't cope, this small inconspicuous little box would bleep and tell me that I had another five urgent things to deal with. Of course I was unaware of all of this on that first innocent evening. Instead, I had a naïve excitement that I was finally considered important enough to have my own pager and that it might actually go off. I had been practising how I should best answer it:

'Hello, it's Dr Daniels, vascular surgical house officer.'

That's right, my first job was as the junior in the vascular surgery team. I didn't really know what vascular surgery was, but I liked the sound of it. Perhaps I could drop the house officer bit and just answer by saying: 'Hi. Dr Daniels, vascular surgeon.' Hmm, that would sound much more impressive. I could just picture the attractive nurse swooning on the other end of the line.

To my surprise, at about ten minutes past five my pager did go off. I took a deep breath and answered the call: 'Hi. Dr Daniels, vascular surgeon.' There was a sigh from the other end of the telephone. It was my consultant and new boss. 'You are not a vascular surgeon, you are my most junior and least useful helper monkey. Some poor bastard has popped his aorta and I'm going to be in theatre with the registrar all evening trying to fix him. I need you to order us a chicken chow mein, a sweet and sour pork and two egg fried rice. Have them delivered to theatre reception.' The phone went dead. That was it. All those years of study and my first job as a doctor was to order a Chinese takeaway. Consultant surgeons have a wonderful way of ensuring that their junior doctors don't get above themselves.

Over the next hour my pager started going off increasingly

frequently until it built up to what felt like a constant chorus of bleeps. Jobs that would take a few minutes for me to do now, took an hour back then because I was so new and inexperienced. I decided that the cocky doctor role didn't suit me so I went for the pathetic vulnerable new doctor approach. It worked and the nurses soon began to feel sorry for me. They offered to make me tea, showed me the secret biscuit cupboard and helped me find my feet. Just as I was beginning to gain a little confidence, my pager made a frightening sound. Instead of the normal slow, steady bleep there was a stream of quick staccato bleeps followed by the words 'Cardiac arrest Willow ward . . . Cardiac arrest Willow ward.' To my horror, that was the ward that my consultant covered. That meant that I should really be there. I started running. The adrenaline was pumping, my white coat was sailing behind me as I zipped past people in the corridor. I was important. It felt great! Suddenly, as I got closer to Willow ward, a terrifying thought dawned on me, 'Oh my God. What if I'm the first doctor there!!!! I've only ever resuscitated a rubber dummy in training exercises. I've never had to do the real thing.' To my left was the gents' toilet. Doubts began to race through my head. 'Perhaps I could just nip in there and hide for a bit. I can reappear in a few minutes once the cavalry has arrived.' It was tempting, but I bravely decided to keep on running and meet my fate.

Lying in a bed was a frail old lady with her pyjamas ripped open and her torso exposed. She was grey and lifeless and I can remember her ribs protruding out of her chest wall. A couple of nurses were frantically running around looking for oxygen and the patient's notes, while another nurse was doing chest compressions. To my relief, a remarkably relaxed-looking medical registrar was standing at the head of the bed and calmly taking charge. A monitor was set up and it was clear even to me that the wiggly lines on the screen meant that the patient needed to be shocked. A few other doctors soon turned up and I was pretty much a spectator as they expertly performed a few rounds of CPR (cardiopulmonary resuscitation) followed by a set of shocks. It was all very dramatic but the woman didn't seem to be making any signs of a revival. Thinking that I had managed to escape my first cardiac arrest as an onlooker only, I began to consider sneaking away, aware of how many mundane jobs were waiting for me to be done on other wards. Unfortunately, the relaxed-looking registrar spotted me and called me forward. 'This one's not coming back; shall we let the house officer have a go with the defibrillator?' I had just done my CPR training and it was all still clear in my mind. This was my big moment. For some reason, I had it in my head that if it was me who shocked her, she would suddenly come round. What a great story that would be, I thought as I stepped up to the bed. The one thing that the instructors had really emphasised in the resuscitation training was the importance of safety. I had to make sure that all the doctors, nurses and oxygen masks were clear of the bed before shocking the patient. I stepped up and took the paddles. Lifting them out of the machine I carefully placed them on the woman's chest. Looking all around me, I started the drill: 'Oxygen away, head clear, feet clear, charging to 360, shocking at 360.'

BANG. My adrenaline had been pumping but I hadn't expected that. I had stayed on my feet but had been thrown backwards with a jolt. That never happened with the dummies. I must have been looking slightly dazed and the registrar glanced over at me with faint amusement. 'You've electrocuted yourself, you prat.' Unfortunately, he was right. I had checked closely to make sure that the bed was clear of bystanders before I gave the electric shock, but I hadn't realised that on running to the ward, I had shoved my stethoscope into the pocket of my white coat and as I was leaning over the patient, the nicely conductive metal tubes had been lying on the patient's left hand.

As if to rub salt in the wound, my first pathetic effort at resuscitation led the woman to go straight into asystole (flatlining) and the registrar called it a day. The correct thing to have done would have been to report my electrocution as a critical incident and give me a bit of a check-over, but instead the registrar just disappeared off the ward chuckling to himself. I had made his night and he called me 'Sparky' for the rest of my six-month spell at the hospital. I was left to carry on with the boring jobs on the ward and by the following morning everyone had heard of my disastrous first night. Perhaps it was an early indicator that I was better suited to the slightly less dramatic world of general practice.

Jargon

At my secondary school I was known as Benny Big Nose. Not the most charming of nicknames, but nevertheless a beautifully simple and succinct summary of my name and most prominent facial feature. I sometimes wish medicine could be as straightforward. Why do we use long-winded medical jargon to describe something rather simple?

Purulent nasal discharge – snot; viral upper respiratory tract infection – a cold; infective gastroenteritis – the shits; strong urinary odour – stinks of piss.

One reason for medical jargon is so that we doctors can write something in the notes that if the patient were to read, they wouldn't take offence and complain. There was a time a few years back when patients had no right at all to see their own medical notes. I was recently looking through the old paper notes of one retired farmer and the sole entry for 1973 was 'Patient smells of pig shit.' How beautifully jargon free.

When I first qualified, I loved all the medical jargon. I felt that it made us sound clever and elite and I got off on the fact that I could have a chat with a fellow medic on the train. However, it only takes an interaction with someone who uses jargon that you don't understand to realise how annoying it can be. Current letters from our managers at the PCT (Primary Care Trust) have just this effect on me. What do phrases like 'performance-based target strategies' and 'competence managed commissioning' mean. They certainly don't seem to bear any relevance to my daily routine of listening to people's health grumbles and trying to make them feel a bit better.

Patients are always happiest if you skip the jargon and say it how it is. I find that replacing the phrase 'stage-four renal impairment' with 'knackered kidneys' or 'mitotic growth' with 'cancer' is generally appreciated. We all like to have things explained in terms we can understand and I just wish that NHS managers would write me letters in a language that I could comprehend.

It was Darren Mills who first named me Benny Big Nose. The last I heard, he was spending some well-deserved time at Her Majesty's pleasure. His straightforward and direct manner seemed to get him in trouble from the teachers and later the police. However, Darren, if you're out there, I'd like to say thank you for teaching me the valuable lesson of saying it how it is. You usually don't cause as much offence as you think you might and most people will appreciate your honesty.

Proud to work for the NHS

One weekend I was doing a locum shift in A&E and saw a middle-aged German couple who had been involved in a car accident. They had been on a driving holiday around the UK and had crashed their car into a ditch. Fortunately, they weren't severely hurt but an ambulance was with them within ten minutes and the paramedics gave some basic first aid before ferrying them to hospital. They were then seen by me and I organised some X-rays to make sure that the man didn't have any neck injuries and to confirm a suspected dislocation of one of the woman's fingers. The man's neck X-ray was fine and I injected some local anaesthetic into the woman's finger and popped the dislocated joint back into place. The healthcare assistant got them a cup of tea and a sandwich each and one of the nurses then cleaned and dressed a few of their cuts and scratches. Finally, the receptionist let them use her phone to call their car hire firm and organise a taxi back to their hotel.

As I let them know that they were free to go, the German man got his wallet out and tried to give me his Visa card. I explained that he didn't have to pay me so he then started giving me his address so that he could be billed at home. I literally had to spend ten minutes convincing him that the treatment he had received was free of charge. 'But everyone has been so good to us,' he protested.

'I wouldn't have got any better treatment back home. Why do you British spend so much time complaining about your health service?' It was one of those moments where I simply felt an overwhelming pride to be a part of the NHS. Of course, there are days when I spend a lot of time apologising for the inadequacies of the NHS, but overall I still believe that if you are genuinely unwell or have an accident, there aren't many places on the planet where you would get a better service.

Sitting around with a bunch of GPs recently, I was surprised by how many thought that there should be a charge to be seen in A&E or by a GP. The general consensus was that £5 would be just enough to keep out some of the time-wasters and make people think twice before pitching up to see us. I have to say I couldn't disagree more. I appreciate that the NHS isn't free because we pay for it with our taxes, but it is free at the point of delivery and I feel that is something fundamentally vital in maintaining some of the original ideals of Nye Bevan and the other founders of the NHS. A charge would keep away some of the more vulnerable people who needed our help most and suddenly change the dynamic and mindset of the patients who would now be paying directly for our services.

Drug reps

Sixteen tablets of a supermarket's own brand ibuprofen cost just 35p, while 16 tablets of Neurofen cost £1.99. This is strange to believe considering they really are exactly the same medicine. The drug company that makes Neurofen uses clever advertising and packaging to convince us to pay over five times more money than we need to.

Drug companies are very good at overcharging us for medicine. In the world of prescription drugs, millions of pounds are wasted by the NHS because doctors prescribe expensive ones when they could be prescribing much cheaper versions of exactly the same medicines. How do the pharmaceutical companies hoodwink us into doing that? Again, it is all about marketing. Young and attractive drug reps come and promote their drugs, while buying us lunch or even taking us out for dinner at posh restaurants. They feed us biased information on why we should use their more expensive medicine and give us free pens and mugs sporting their brand. (There are now much stricter rules than there used to be about how much drug reps can spend on us doctors. For example, the free gifts that they give us now have to be under the value of £5 and when drug reps take us all out for a slap-up meal, there has to be an 'educational' component to the evening rather than a completely uninterrupted session of good food and expensive wine. The drug companies' all-expenses-paid trips to 'conferences' in the Caribbean have stopped, too.)

I used to attend the lunches and dinners. As I pocketed the free gifts and scoffed down the expensive nosh, I convinced myself that we doctors were too 'savvy' to be influenced by colourful flip charts and pretty smiles. The pharmaceutical industry, of course, knows that this isn't the case. A few hundred quid taking some GPs out for dinner is peanuts compared to the money they can make if one or two of us start prescribing their drug.

In the USA, pharmaceutical companies employ ex-American football players and cheerleaders to sell their products. Doctors are suckers for a pretty face like everyone else. The attractive female reps are sent to sell their products to the predominantly male surgical consultants, while the pretty-boy male reps sell to the more female-dominated obstetric and paediatric departments. Fortunately in this country, our retired sports stars tend to fall ungracefully into alcoholism and gambling addiction rather than trying to sell us overpriced medicines. I can't imagine even the most star-struck doctor being convinced to prescribe an anti-depressant promoted by Gazza or a painkiller endorsed by Vinnie Jones.

As well as constant pressure from drug reps, GPs also face resistance from patients when trying to change medication. Whenever I can, I try to switch my patients from the more expensive medicines to the cheaper ones that do the same thing. Unfortunately, this can be very unpopular with patients. Often they get used to a certain packet and tablet colour and no amount of persuasion will convince them to switch. One elderly lady once stormed into my surgery furious that I had changed her medicine:

'You told me that the new medicine was the same as the old one!'

'Yes that's right, Mrs Goodson – same medicine, but different name.'

'Well, I know that's nonsense because when I try to flush these tablets down the toilet, they don't float like the old ones did.'

Drug reps have the cheek to claim that they are helping to educate us by updating us on the latest scientific research. This is, of course, nonsense as their only interest is flogging their drug and earning a commission if prescribing rates of their drug increase on their patch. They give ruthlessly one-sided presentations that show their pill to be wonderful and ignore the parts of the research that don't paint their drug so favourably.

Having finally realised that I will only ever get biased information from the pharmaceutical industry, I now refuse to see any drug reps. They hover around the reception desk like prowling hyenas, only to be batted away by the fierce receptionist. Not having the time or inclination to read all the medical journals myself, I rely on the local NHS pharmacist to keep me up to date with the new medications on the market. She is a fount of knowledge on all the latest scientific research and doesn't work on commission. Like me, she has the best interest of the patient at heart, while also keeping half an eye on the NHS budget. There really is no such thing as a free lunch and so I'll pay for my own, thanks.

Mr Tipton, the paedophile

I had been asked to go on a home visit to see a patient I hadn't met before. Mr Tipton was in his fifties and complaining of having diarrhoea. There was some kind of gastric flu going round at the time, but normally a 50-year-old could manage the squits without needing a doctor's visit.

As I skimmed through his notes, there was one item that stood out. In between entries for a slightly high blood pressure reading and a chesty cough was 'imprisonment for child sex offences'. Mr Tipton was a paedophile. There were no gory details of his offences but he had spent six years in prison and had only recently been released.

Mr Tipton lived in Somersby House. Despite the pleasant sounding name, Somersby House is a shithole, a 17-storey 1960s tower block as grey and intimidating on the inside as it is on the outside. As I waited an eternity for the lift to climb the 17 floors, I wondered if the strong smell of stale urine was coming from one of my fellow passengers or the building as a whole. The grey-faced natives eyed me suspiciously; I was looking conspicuously out of place in my shiny shoes and matching shirt and tie. A mental note was made to keep a spare tracksuit and baseball cap in the car to disguise myself on my next visit.

I was annoyed and ashamed by how uncomfortable I felt in Somersby House. When I started medical school I felt distinctly 'street'. While most of my compatriots were privately educated somewhere in the Home Counties, I went to an inner city comprehensive. Why was I feeling so bloody middle class? Medical school had not only desensitised me to death and suffering, it had also turned me into a snob.

I finally got to Mr Tipton's flat. After several minutes of knocking on the door and shouting through the letter box, he finally answered. Walking unsteadily with the aid of a Zimmer frame, he was wearing a filthy grey vest and nothing else. As I followed him into his flat, his bare buttocks were wasted and smeared with dried faeces. The flat was like nothing I had ever seen. There were beer cans and cigarette butts in their hundreds. The floor was brown and sticky and I tried desperately to manoeuvre myself down the corridor without touching anything.

It was the bedroom that was truly shocking. It transpired that Mr Tipton had been pretty much bedridden for the last few days with a bad back and he hadn't been able to make it to the toilet when the diarrhoea struck. There was shit everywhere! His bed consisted of a bare mattress and a coverless duvet. Both were covered in an unfeasible quantity of faeces that looked both old and recent. There were cider bottles filled with his urine and an empty takeaway wrapper covered in vomit. It was truly grim. Amazingly, as we arrived in his room, Mr Tipton calmly laid himself back on the mattress and pulled the shitty duvet over him. I donned some gloves and half-heartedly had a prod of his belly. I made a few token comments about letting viruses take their course and then fled.

I gave social services a call and asked them to go round to do an 'urgent assessment of his care needs'. In other words: 'Come round and clear up this shit.' I made it very clear to the social worker that I didn't think that Mr Tipton required any more medical input as I had done a thorough assessment and diagnosed a self-limiting viral gastroenteritis. I hoped she wouldn't see through my bullshit and realise that I was, in fact, just desperately trying to wash my hands of Mr Tipton and make him someone else's problem.

On my drive back to the surgery, I wondered why Mr Tipton had allowed himself to lie in his own shit for the last three days. Perhaps he was in some way allowing himself to be punished for his awful crimes. Or was it just that he had a dodgy back and couldn't get to the phone? Maybe there was simply no one else whom he knew he could call on. I often visit lonely, isolated people for whom the GP is their only contact with the outside world. Normally, I reach out to these abandoned people with some compassion and kindness. Why hadn't I done this for Mr Tipton? Reflecting back, I know that my knowledge of Mr Tipton's crimes influenced my behaviour towards him. Although I couldn't have offered him much more as a doctor, I could have offered him a great deal more as a human. The Hippocratic oath tells us that it is not our place to judge our patients but only to treat each one with impartiality and compassion. I think I agree with this in principle but offering kindness and empathy to a paedophile covered in shit isn't always easy.

Average day

I sometimes think that people have an odd preconception of what makes up the typical day for a GP. These are the exact patients that I saw one morning, a wet Tuesday in November in a typical practice somewhere in the south of England. None of the consultations are outlandish or exciting enough to deserve their own chapter, but they are a very typical reflection of a GP's average morning.

1. A seven-year-old boy having tummy aches. Mum was very worried, as her nephew had had a kidney transplant at a similar age. The tummy aches only occurred on mornings before school and after finally managing to keep Mum quiet for a few minutes, I asked the lad a few questions and he admitted that another boy was bullying him at school. Mum left the surgery and stormed straight up to the school.

2. A very nice woman in her thirties with six-month-old twins. She was finding it all a bit much and was very tearful. She did actually have symptoms of postnatal depression and was worried that it could be affecting her relationship with her children. We had a long chat about possible options, including counselling and antidepressants. She would be coming back to see me in a couple

of days to let me know what she had decided to do and so I could see how she was getting on. I also wrote a letter to the health visitor to see what other support she could get.

3. A 60-year-old woman worried about the appearance of yellow lumps around her eyes. I explained they looked like cholesterol deposits. She told me that there was no point in her having a cholesterol test, as she refused to take any Western medicine and therefore wouldn't take any cholesterol-lowering medication even if her cholesterol was high. She was also convinced that her diet couldn't be any healthier than it already was. I told her about risks of having a stroke or a heart attack but I was happy that she was entitled to make her own informed choice not to have the test. I made sure I documented this carefully so she couldn't come back and sue me at a later date.

4. A very nice woman in her fifties with breast cancer. She had chemotherapy and radiotherapy over the summer and thankfully her cancer seemed to be in remission. She told me that she lay in bed at night and every time she felt the slightest tingle in her fingers or an ache in her leg, she was convinced that it was the sign of her cancer coming back. We had a long chat and I tried to reassure her that her fears were normal and understandable. I put her in touch with a cancer support group.

5. A middle-aged woman with a slightly sore knee for two days, which was getting better. I went through the motions of examining her but everything looked normal. I couldn't really work out what she was expecting me to do for her. She seemed happy enough with my reassurance.

6.   An 80-year-old man who had had some diarrhoea over the
     weekend, which had since settled. He actually wanted to talk
     about the current legal wrangling he was having with his
     niece who was trying to evict him from his family home. I
     listened for about 15 minutes but was already running very late
     so had to cut him short and move on to the next patient.

7.   A 30-year-old woman with a cold. She had come in specifically for
     antibiotics and she made this clear from the start. I examined her
     fully and then explained in much detail why antibiotics weren't
     going to help her as she had a viral infection. She was very insis-
     tent that she wanted antibiotics as she had an important work
     presentation to do on Friday! She was not happy at all when I
     refused to prescribe her antibiotics.

8.   A 40-year-old man involved in a mild car accident over the
     weekend. He had some very mild muscle aches in his neck but
     nothing that needed to be seen by a doctor. He was only here for
     insurance purposes in case he decided to make a claim at a later
     date. I was slightly annoyed that he had used up an urgent slot
     for this. This is an example of one of the few instances where I
     feel we should charge patients to be seen.

9.   A fairly straightforward tennis elbow. However, the man was a self-
     employed mechanic so when I advised him to rest his arm, he gave
     me a resigned smile and said, 'I'd love to, mate, but who's going to
     run my garage?' I referred him to a physio and advised painkillers.

10. A three-month-old baby with a cold. Very cute. She was absolutely
     fine and smiled throughout my examination. A smiling baby always
     helps lift my spirits, especially halfway through a busy morning.

11. A very anxious woman who was convinced she had had an allergic reaction to her latest blood pressure medication. She had a history of lots of unusual medication allergies. Perhaps they were genuine allergies or perhaps there was a degree of hysteria. She was far too frightening for me to argue with so I stopped the medication and agreed to try yet another one.

12. A woman in her late sixties with a cough and breathlessness. She thought she had a chest infection but on closer inspection it looked to be actually due to a build-up of fluid in her lungs because of problems with her heart. I spent some time explaining the likely diagnosis and started her on some new medications and also ordered various tests.

13. A patient didn't turn up – frustrating, as many patients phoned this morning wanting an appointment but were told that there were none available. I have to admit that it was a relief for me in some ways. I was running late by now so I had the chance to catch up a little bit.

14. A very odd case. A 38-year-old woman came in to see me. She was seven weeks pregnant and had been trying to get pregnant for years. Previously, she had been seen in the infertility clinic and had had two miscarriages. She told me that she wanted an abortion because she had felt so unwell since becoming pregnant and couldn't cope with the symptoms. It was also a bad time for her to be pregnant. She had just been to the hospital for a scan which showed a normal pregnancy so far. She was flying next Thursday, so wanted the abortion before then. I'm sure there was something she wasn't telling me. My suspicion was that the pregnancy was the result of an affair but I'm just

guessing. I referred her to the specialist clinic and I know that they do a long and detailed assessment prior to considering an abortion.

15. A 17-year-old girl seen with her mum. She had a long history of being seen by lots of specialists. Mum was convinced that her daughter had 'never been well due to a weak immune system', although all tests have been normal. She was being schooled at home. All a bit weird and I wasn't keen on being dragged in too deeply as I was not her normal doctor. I looked through the notes and saw that despite having apparently 'never been well', she did manage to get herself pregnant last year and have an abortion and was also recently seen in A&E after getting into a drunken fight outside a pub. Hmmm. They just wanted a repeat prescription of her normal medication, so that was easy enough.

16. An 80-year-old man who arrived 20 minutes late and couldn't remember why he'd come to see me. He lived alone and drove everywhere. I suggested that we assessed his memory but he refused. I also suggested that if his memory was poor, maybe he should stop driving until he had an assessment from the DVLA. He refused this as well. I decided to contact the DVLA myself. It was a break in confidentiality and his driving might have been fine, but if he killed someone in an accident . . . I wrote the letter.

I finished the morning surgery late and grabbed a sandwich before rushing off to do a couple of visits:

Visit 1. A 78-year-old man who had had a mini stroke the night before. He had had 11 previous mini strokes and was on all the right medication to control his blood pressure, keep his cholesterol low and thin his blood, etc. He had recovered fully since the previous night and my visit wasn't really necessary medically, but his wife was anxious and I spent 20 minutes reassuring her that she was doing all the right things and she thanked me repeatedly for coming out to see them.

Visit 2. A 57-year-old man who couldn't get out of bed that morning. He was previously fairly well. Initially, I thought he was being a bit precious but then I noticed that the whites of his eyes were a bit yellow (jaundice) and on examining his abdomen, found he had a big liver. Unfortunately, my gut instinct was that he probably had cancer. He asked me what I thought was wrong and I said that I thought there were all sorts of possible causes and I wouldn't like to commit until he had had a scan. Once back at the surgery, I make a referral to get him seen urgently by the bowel and liver specialist. Should I have said I thought he had cancer? I wouldn't want to worry him unnecessarily if he just had gallstones or something completely benign.

So there we are. That was my morning. There were also a few extra phone calls and prescriptions to sign. The nurse popped in inbetween patients to ask me a few questions and I had to dictate some letters and sign some forms. I had a quick cup of tea and got myself ready for the afternoon surgery.

That was exactly what I did that morning. I have no idea if that fits your expectation of an average GP's morning but there it is and probably fairly typical for most GPs. It was, perhaps, unusual in its absence of drug-abuse problems and sick-note requests, but that was probably mostly because the practice was in quite a middle-class area. Fortunately for me, I found the morning interesting, challenging and rewarding. It was a typical morning, but would still be completely different from yesterday and tomorrow.

Tara

'Doctor, you fucked up my medication again. That antidepressant you gave me was fucking useless and I need another sick note.'

Tara is taxing; we call them 'heart-sink' patients. When she walks into my consulting room my heart sinks to the floor and I often find myself hoping that it will stop altogether.

I try to view Tara with compassion. She is a vulnerable adult who grew up in an abusive, socially deprived family and she needs support and patience. The problem is that when running late on a Friday afternoon, my empathy is often overtaken by frustration and annoyance. I'm ashamed to admit it but rather than offer the time, patience and support Tara requires, I often find myself wishing I was somewhere else.

I sort out Tara's medication and then ponder what to write on the sick note. Tara is 25 and has never worked. She doesn't have a physical disability or a neat diagnosis to put on the dotted line. She isn't depressed or psychotic, although she has seen a multitude of psychiatrists, psychologists and counsellors. The only firm diagnosis Tara has ever been given is 'borderline personality disorder'.

I find the concept of personality disorders difficult, but my limited understanding is that someone with this diagnosis has a personality that doesn't really fit in with the rest of society and they struggle to cope with all aspects of modern life. Most would agree that our personalities arise from a combination of nature and nurture, but in the case of Tara, growing up with an extreme lack of anything that could be called nurture is the principal problem. People with borderline personality disorders tend to act like stroppy teenagers. They often only see things in black and white and fly off the handle easily. They don't have a particularly good idea of who they are and always seem to fall into stormy, damaging relationships. They have low self-esteem and often self-harm as a way of expressing their frustrations with life.

Stroppy teenagers grow up, but people with borderline personality disorders don't. They struggle to cope with the adult world and require a huge amount of support and understanding from those around them. Despite being able to rationalise all this, I still find my consultations with Tara madly frustrating and I would love to prescribe her a twice daily kick up the arse. I am not proud that I feel like that about my most regular patient but I know that she also brings out similar feelings in the other doctors at the practice. Some smart-arse psychoanalyst would tell me that my ambivalence towards Tara is a reflection of my own feelings of failure in my inability to help her. I'm sure that is true but I can't help but wish she didn't come and see me quite so often.

I do occasionally have a 'Conservative moment' and feel righteous about why a physically fit 25-year-old has never worked and probably never will, but you only have to spend a few minutes with Tara to realise that her chaotic existence just wouldn't cope with work. When she doesn't like something, she either cuts herself or flies into a rage. She is a mess emotionally and no employer in their right mind would want her working for them. She has had input from all sorts of well-meaning and well-funded services over the years, but seeing a supportive social worker, health visitor, GP or psychiatrist for 15 minutes a week hasn't managed to counter-act the harm caused by 25 years of growing up in an abusive and damaging family.

Sometimes I worry that doctors write off patients with person-ality disorders too quickly. Some people go so far as to claim that it is a 'made-up' diagnosis that doctors put upon patients with mental health issues that are challenging and don't fit tidily into any other diagnosis. There is no pill that cures a personality disorder so we label the person as a lost cause and withdraw all help and support. This seems a shame given that many of the chronic diseases we do treat can't be cured. We don't give up on our patients with diabetes because they can't be cured. Instead, we do our best to control their symptoms as best we can and try to work with them to give them the best possible quality of life.

After a bit of reflection, I promise myself that I'll be a bit nicer to Tara next time she visits. I'll try to listen harder and be more supportive. I'll give her more of my time and won't rush her out the door. Maybe she'll open up a little more to me? Maybe she won't even notice? At least I will feel like a slightly nicer doctor for a few minutes.

Sex in the surgery

According to a study in France, 1 in 10 male GPs questioned have had a relationship with a patient and 1 in 12 admitted to having actively tried to seduce a patient. One French doctor reportedly stated, 'It is obvious that some patients like us and we are not made of wood.' I have to say, I was quite surprised by the results of this study. When compared to the general population, I would say that my doctor friends are probably on the lower end of the scale when it comes to morals and good behaviour. Despite this, I can honestly say that I don't think that any have had a relationship with a patient or even considered it. As medical students and junior doctors, we got up to all sorts of debauchery both sexual and otherwise, but somehow having sex with a patient never really figured. It is perhaps one of the few taboo subjects that remain among us. We will happily sit round in the pub competing to see who had made the worst medical error as a junior doctor, or recalling past drunken sexual adventures with the unfortunate student nurses who had fallen foul of our charms, but even admitting to finding a patient attractive just doesn't happen.

When I started my medical career, my non-medical friends seemed to imagine that I would have all sorts of saucy 'Carry on Doctor' moments with beautiful female patients. They were disappointed when I explained that as a hospital doctor, I rarely had a patient under 65. My days were spent looking at fungating leg ulcers and sputum samples, rather than pulling splinters out of the behinds of young Barbara Windsor lookalikes.

Since moving to general practice, I do have young female patients. There is also more of an intimacy that develops between doctor and patient. It is less about the proximity of the physical examination, but more about the openness and intimacy of the consultation. The patient is able to disclose their deepest, darkest feelings and fears, often revealing secrets that they wouldn't divulge to their closest friends or family. It is part of the privilege of being a doctor and it is our job to listen and be supportive. Often the GP might be the only person in an individual's life who does listen to them without judgement or criticism and it is this that can make us the object of attraction.

In my career as a doctor, I can think of three female patients who have made a pass at me. One was a lonely single mum, one was a lonely teenager and the third was a lonely foreign-exchange student. They all visited me regularly and offloaded their fears and worries. I sat and listened when no one else would; I nodded and made supportive noises; I was encouraging and made positive suggestions as I handed them tissues to mop up their tears. Vulnerable people can mistake this for affection. It is easy for a lonely person to forget that I'm being paid to listen to them. These three women fell for me because, unlike in a real relationship, the baggage was offloaded in one direction only. I didn't get to talk about my regrets and fears. I wasn't allowed to display my needy and vulnerable side. If my love-struck patients had to hear all my shit, I'm sure my desirability would have quickly dissolved.

I do care about my patients and I try my hardest to empathise, but ultimately my patients are not my friends or family members and once they leave my room, I move on to the next patient and problem. This may seem cold and callous, but if doctors got emotionally involved with all our patients and their unhappiness, our work would consume us and send us spiralling into depression ourselves. This does happen to some doctors. We call it 'burn out' and it doesn't benefit doctor or patient.

The Hippocratic oath states: In every house where I come, I will enter only for the good of my patients, keeping myself far from all intentional ill-doing and all seduction and especially from the pleasures of love with women or with men.

Many people, including at least 1 in 10 French doctors, probably feel that this is out of date and that consenting sex between two adults shouldn't be frowned upon just because one happens to be the other's doctor. I have to say that I agree with the Greek fella in this case. He clearly recognised the uniqueness of the doctor–patient bond and the vulnerability of the patient in this relationship. A sexual liaison that forms in this environment can never be equal, as the doctor will always hold a position of power and trust. In general, the medical profession's governing bodyagrees with this and in the UK, quite rightly, doctors are still in a whole heap of the brown stuff if they have a relationship with a patient.

The elderly

My first patient of the morning is Mr A. He is 35 and has a sore ear. He only comes to the doctor about twice a year. I look inside and it is blocked with wax. During his ten-minute appointment I have explained the diagnosis, had a bit of a chat and sent him on his way with some ear drops. The medication is cheap, he gets better and I feel happy as a doctor that I have cured my patient. I am also running on time and know that I will get to the coffee before all the nice biscuits have been eaten by the receptionists.

My second patient of the morning is Mrs B. She is 87 and has come in with painful legs, a sore back, dizzy spells and some breathlessness. It takes her nearly half of her appointment time to shuffle in from the waiting room and take off her four cardigans. She is lonely and socially isolated and really wants to chat. She is a bit forgetful and not very good at giving me a clear story about what hurts when and where. She is already on a multitude of drugs, which she often forgets to take. After a long, disjointed consultation, she departs after 30 minutes without any of her symptoms really being treated and leaves me feeling like I'm not a very good doctor. She will be back next week with a new list of problems. My subsequent patients are annoyed because I am running late and by the time I get to coffee, I am left with a couple of broken, stale digestives.

One of the joys of being a GP is having a close and supportive relationship with elderly patients, but they really do take up the lion's share of our workload. By definition, the ageing process means that as we get older, more and more things go irreversibly wrong until we finally die. This can be quite hard for both the doctor and the patient to accept. Of course, there are fantastic sprightly 90-year-olds who never visit the doctor and moping 20-years-olds who spend their lives in my waiting room. But generally speaking, the older you get, the more you see your GP.

Treating elderly people with multiple complex medical and social problems is one of the more challenging areas of our work. The goal is to work as part of a team to maintain the person's dignity and autonomy, while pacifying anxious relatives and navigating through the bureaucracy that is the NHS and social services. Elderly patients are often fantastically appreciative and working with them can be extremely rewarding. Having said all that, it is bloody hard work!

I worked once in a city practice in a young trendy part of town. There simply weren't many elderly people who lived there. I saw more patients in less time and didn't do any home visits. I had less disease targets to worry about because few of my young patients had chronic conditions such as heart disease and diabetes. I sat in a trendy coffee shop during my lunch hour, while my GP colleagues around the country traipsed round nursing homes and arranged home helps and hospital admissions. My job was certainly easier but also less rewarding and less interesting.

I recently read that Harold Shipman's murders were motiveless. I don't think they were. Most GPs could think of several frail, vulnerable elderly patients who take up a lot of their time. Shipman murdered his. One of the hardest parts of being a GP is taking care of elderly people wanting help for untreatable degenerative diseases. Most of us find that listening and offering some practical support and advice is the best we can do and actually very much appreciated. Shipman clearly viewed things differently and felt it was his right to murder his elderly frail patients. I imagine he enjoyed the power but I also think he was motivated by reducing his workload.

Bums

Intimate examinations can be awkward for both doctor and patient. Fortunately, a good explanation and reassurance from the doctor can make the whole procedure a lot less difficult. When the patient doesn't speak very much English, the situation can be that bit more uncomfortable. This was the scenario I faced with Olga, a young Bulgarian woman who came to see me.

'Pain in bottom, Doctor,' she said in a very broad Eastern European accent.

I began to ask a few questions about what sort of pain it was. Was it related to going to the toilet? Was there any blood in the poo? These are all the normal questions that would usually give a doctor a fairly good idea of what the diagnosis might be. The problem was that each question was met with blank confusion. Olga had clearly found out how to say 'pain in bottom' but was unable to understand any word I said. Despite a brilliant attempt on my part to mime diarrhoea and constipation using a mixture of diagrams, sound effects and facial expressions, I was getting nowhere. Feeling completely useless, the only option I had left was to examine her. I motioned towards the couch and mouthed out the word 'EXAMINATION' very slowly and loudly. Olga seemed to understand, so I pulled round the curtain to give her some privacy as she undressed.

As those of you who have had the misfortune to have had your bottom examined by the doctor will know, we generally expect you to drop your trousers, jump up on the bed, pull your knees up to your chest and lie on your side facing away from the doctor. I usually have a blanket handy so the patient can remain covered until the examination itself takes place. Normally, the whole ordeal is quick and relatively painless – well, painless for me, anyway. Unfortunately, it would appear that things are done slightly differently in Bulgaria. I pulled back the curtain to find Olga naked from the waist down leaning over the couch with her bottom pointing to the ceiling. 'No no, you need to be up on the bed!' I cried. 'ON THE BED,' I repeated slowly and loudly. I pulled the curtain across again and after a few polite moments went back in. This time Olga was on all fours on top of the couch still with her bum pointing up in the air. After much gesticulating and loud slow explanations, I was still no closer to having Olga in a position in which I could examine her. I motioned for her to get off the bed and got on myself lying in the correct position. 'LIKE THIS, YOU SEE.' I was lying curled up on the bed while my half-naked patient was standing beside me still looking very puzzled. It was a moment that I was very glad wasn't interrupted by a receptionist bringing in a cup of tea.

I did finally manage to examine Olga's bottom, only to find nothing unusual at all. In theory I should have done a rectal examination as well, but poor Olga had faced enough already and inserting my finger up her back passage without her really being able to understand my explanation of what I was doing seemed a bit unfair, bordering on abuse. I managed to book her in for an appointment another time with an interpreter present but she didn't turn up, possibly having somewhat lost faith in me.

I recall another difficult rectal examination back when I was an A&E doctor. An elderly lady called Ethel had been brought in by her husband, Lionel, because of her having some tummy pains and bleeding from her anus. Ethel herself was quite demented and also very deaf. Lionel was a retired vicar and now caring for Ethel full time at home.

After taking a history from Lionel and feeling Ethel's tummy, I needed to do a rectal examination. It was important to make sure that there wasn't a blockage in the rectum causing her symptoms. 'I'm going to need to examine your rectum, Ethel.' 'You what, love? I can't hear you.' 'I need to put a digit up your back passage, Ethel,' I say again a bit louder and into her good ear. 'What's he saying, eh?' 'I'M GOING TO HAVE TO PUT A FINGER UP YOUR BOTTOM.' This time I was shouting at the top of my lungs. It was only a set of curtains that separated us from the rest of the A&E department and, as you can imagine, curtains aren't particularly soundproof. The entirety of the A&E department was now aware of Ethel's impending rectal examination but, unfortunately, Ethel wasn't. Her confusion was such that she couldn't really comprehend what I was doing or why. Despite my best efforts to put her at ease, she was getting increasingly agitated. I put on a pair of gloves, moved her into as comfortable a position as possible and gently eased my right index finger into her anus. Suddenly, there was an almighty shriek. 'Oooh, Lionel. Stop it, Lionel. You know I don't like it that way. If you've got to put it in, at least put it in around the front.' Poor Lionel was standing outside the cubicle in full view of all the patients and staff who were trying to hold back their giggles. He looked very embarrassed as he made his way back into the cubicle.

Julia

Julia was young, attractive and articulate.

'I need you to section my boyfriend Andy. He's completely mad and unreasonable and yesterday he smashed up my moped for no reason.'

I wasn't expecting that one.

'Your boyfriend doesn't sound very nice but we aren't going to be able to section him.'

'But he's mad! It wasn't just any moped. It was my twenty-first birthday present. I drove it everywhere. It was my most precious possession! He knew that!'

I was tempted to explain that there wasn't a special subclause in the Mental Health Act that allowed us to section people if the moped they smashed up was a very special birthday present. I held back and instead explained how a person would need to have a mental disorder and pose a risk of harming themselves or others before they could be sectioned.

'He is a risk to me. He beats me up!' Julia then proceeded to lift her shirt to reveal an impressive array of bruises on her torso.

'Why don't you leave him? There is a local domestic violence support group. Perhaps I could –'

Julia interrupted me. 'He needs me. He says he would kill himself if I left him and I couldn't have that on my conscience for the rest of my life. He needs help and all you're telling me to do is leave him. He was abused as a child and so was his mum. His whole family is fucked up. I'm all he's got.'

I wasn't sure where to go from here. From the outside it seemed so straightforward. Leave, run away, start again. Julia had a lot going for her. She could have a whole new life. It clearly isn't this straightforward as there are thousands of women like Julia who don't leave or run away or start again. I would never really understand the complexities of Julia's violent relationship but one thing was very clear. When she said that Andy had nobody else, what she was really saying was that she didn't have anyone else. She was alone and, however difficult and abusive her relationship was, she clearly felt that it was all she had.

I was feeling guilty now. Initially, I hadn't really been taking Julia seriously. I had thought that she wanted her boyfriend sectioned because they had had a tiff. It was now clear that things were more complex. Deep down Julia knew that I wasn't going to section Andy but she was crying out for help and somehow it was me who was expected to provide this help. At medical school I had learnt about the role of mitochondrial antibodies in primary biliary cirrhosis and the parasympathetic nerve distribution to the salivary glands. It wasn't the greatest preparation for dealing with a vulnerable desperate woman who got beaten up every day by the man who supposedly loved her. Regardless of my lack of training, at that moment I was all she had and I had to do my best.

'If you leave him and he harms himself, that's not your fault.'

'Is that the best you can do? He needs help.'

Andy was a patient at another practice and I had never met him. I couldn't really speculate what he needed but psychotherapy is usually our get-out clause when faced with a difficult psychological issue that is complex and not fixed with a tablet.

'Maybe psychotherapy would help Andy?'

Julia looked hopeful until I explained that there was a two-year wait for psychotherapy in this town.

'That's really useful, thanks a lot.'

'You have to leave him,' I said again. I tried to say it with compassion but I really did feel it was her only option. Julia got up, left and slammed the door. I clearly hadn't handled that very well. I had failed again. Would another doctor have handled that better? What would a counsellor have said, or a priest or even bloody Jeremy Kyle? I was not sure if Julia would come back to see me. If she did, maybe next time I'd just listen.

Good doctors

What makes a good doctor? I seem to remember being asked something like this during my medical school interview. The interview panel yawned through my contrived answer that mentioned some naïve nonsense about being caring and good at working in a team. As part of our target-based existence, the patient plays a large role in deciding if we are good doctors or not. The Labour government introduced patient satisfaction questionnaires as part of our performance targets.

During my training year I saw a middle-aged woman with stomach pains. I was very concerned and referred her urgently to the hospital because I thought she might have stomach cancer. She was seen and investigated within a week and turned out to simply have bad indigestion. When the snotty letter came back from the consultant, I was feeling a little red in the face. I had made an inappropriate expensive referral to the hospital and had caused unnecessary anxiety to the patient. I could just imagine the consultant grumbling into his endoscope as he cursed me for adding to his already busy day.

The patient and her husband, however, thought the sun shone out of my arse. 'That wonderful Dr Daniels arranged for me to be seen so quickly.' She bought me a very nice bottle of single malt to say thank you and told anyone who'd listen how fantastic I was. My poor medical judgement earned me a rather nice bottle of whisky and if my patient got to fill in one of the patient satisfaction questionnaires, I'd have been reported as the best doctor in the world.

Most medical practitioners have an idea whether they're being good or bad doctors. On a Friday afternoon when I'm drained and tired, I know that I'm not giving my all. I try my best to remain professional but have to admit that I find it that bit harder to resist inappropriate requests for hospital referrals, sick notes and antibiotics. As GPs, we are supposed to be the 'gatekeepers of the NHS' but sometimes it can feel much easier to leave the gate permanently ajar rather than carefully defend the NHS hospital waiting lists by fending off the worried well. I'm very popular with my patients on a Friday afternoon because they are getting what they want, but I'm not always practising good medicine. Making the patient happy isn't always the same as being a good doctor.

When I started as a GP I was told that it was easy to be a bad GP but hard to be a good one. A good doctor won't prescribe antibiotics for a cold and won't refer every patient with a headache for an expensive MRI scan. A good doctor should also be able to explain to the patient why he's not agreeing to their demands, but sometimes, however hard you try, the patient leaves feeling dissatisfied and the doctor goes home feeling distinctly unpopular. It is a difficult balance to run on time but give each patient adequate individual attention, to allow patient choice but not give in to inappropriate demands, to keep referral rates low but make sure the patients get the expert input they need. I'm still not sure exactly what a good doctor is, but it is certainly more complex than earning a few smiley faces on a government questionnaire.

Connor

'It's my kids, Doctor. They're little fuckers. I can't control 'em no more. Something's gotta be done about it. My youngest, Connor, was brought home by the police the other day.'

'How old is Connor?'

'He's three.'

I rack my brains trying to think what a three-year-old could possibly do to get himself in trouble with the police.

'They caught him putting rubbish through the neighbours' letter boxes.'

'Was he out on his own?' I ask incredulously.

'Oh no, Doctor, Bradley and Kylie was with him, but they was the ones telling him to do it.'

I skim through the notes to see that older siblings Bradley and Kylie are six and seven, respectively.

Mum Kerry is actually very likeable. She is a stereotypical council estate mum. Only 25, but already has three kids with three different men who are all now nowhere to be seen. Life is hard for her and she has very little support. She genuinely wants the best for her kids and really wants help.

Unfortunately for her, the entirety of my knowledge on child behaviour comes from having watched a couple of episodes of

Supernanny on TV. I've never been the sternest of people and given the way my cat walks all over me, I'm probably not the best person to ask about discipline.

'I think he's got that DDHD condition. You know, where they're little shits but it's 'cause there's something wrong with the chemicals in their brain and that.'

I've met lots of parents whose children have had a diagnosis of attention deficit hyperactivity disorder (ADHD). The parents love the label because it now excuses the bad behaviour. The kids run riot round my consulting room, rifling through my sharps bin and using my ophthalmoscope as a hammer. Mum and Dad do nothing to stop them and then say, 'Sorry about the kids, Doc. It's the ADHD – nothing we can do . . . brain chemicals and that.'

I don't disbelieve that ADHD exists but perhaps it has been overdiagnosed in recent years. The main symptoms are lack of concentration, being easily distracted and not being good at listening. I could probably persuade myself that Connor has these symptoms, but I'm not sure that they are related to brain chemicals. I guess some children are more prone to developing these symptoms than others, but in most cases isn't parenting more likely to be the most significant factor rather than a brain disease?

I'm not going to send Kerry's kids to the child psychiatrist. The wait is long and I don't want these children labelled as psychiatrically unwell. I've heard there is a specialist social worker locally who gives individual and group parenting skills classes. Kerry is perfect for her.

Kerry comes back a couple of weeks later to let me know how it went.

'I really like my parenting support worker. She told me I mustn't call 'em little fuckers no more but instead they are good children with some c.h.a.l.l.e.n.g.i.n.g behaviour.'

She goes on to tell me about how she is now rewarding good

behaviour, setting consistent boundaries and using the naughty corner. Hold on a minute, I could have told her that. This parenting adviser must have watched the same episode of *Supernanny* that I saw.

Janine

Janine is nine years old and about 13 stone. She waddles into my room and then Mum waddles in after her. My room feels very small.

'It's her ankles, Doctor. They hurt when she runs at school. She needs a note to say that she can sit out games.'

'Did you fall over or twist your ankle, Janine?' I always try to engage with the child themselves if possible. Janine looks at the floor and then shakes her head. 'How long have they been sore?' Eyes still to the floor, this time I get a shrug.

'Right, let's have a look at these ankles then.' I try to be engaging and smiley, stay positive and encouraging. I prod and poke her ankles and get her to move them around a bit. My examination is a bit of a show most of the time and today is no exception. One look at Janine walking into my room showed me that her ankles were basically normal. I try to make my prodding and poking look like it has purpose, but it is purely a performance for the benefit of Janine and her mum. I want them to think that I am taking them seriously, that I am genuinely looking for some 'underlying ankle pathology'. As I prod away, I try to remember the names of some of the ankle ligaments . . . no joy there. Perhaps I'll just try to remember which is the tibia and which is the fibula . . . no, just confusing myself now.

'Right . . . Well, I can't find any swelling or tenderness in those ankles . . . and she's walking okay . . .' This is the make or break moment . . . How am I going to put this tactfully? I am standing at the top of the diving board but do I have the bottle to make that jump? I could just write the note, prescribe some paracetamol syrup and climb quietly down the ladder. No, Daniels, come on, it's your duty to say something. Right. Here goes. 'Some children find that . . . erm err . . . that being a bit . . . erm . . .' (Say it, Daniels, just say it) '. . . erm overweight can make their joints hurt sometimes.' I had done it. I had jumped!

Janine's mum looks me straight in the eye. Her face looks like a pitbull slowly chewing a wasp. 'It's got nothing to do with her weight,' she says angrily. 'Janine's cousin is as skinny as a rake and she has problems with her ankles, too. It's hereditary.'

What can I say to that? My courageous leap got me nowhere. I belly-flopped painfully. Can I prove that Janine's ankles hurt because she is fat? No. Is Janine's mum going to accept that weight is an issue? No. I either argue on fruitlessly or accept that I am beaten and salvage the few scraps of the patient–doctor relationship that are still intact.

'She can still do swimming!' I shout as they waddle away, sick note and paracetamol prescription already tucked snugly into Mum's handbag. It is a final attempt to redeem myself, but a poor one. I can picture Janine sitting in the changing rooms munching on some crisps while the rest of her class runs around outside. Beneath the many layers of abdominal fat, her pancreas would be slowly preparing itself for a lifetime of insulin resistance and the debilitating symptoms of diabetes that occur as a result. Meanwhile, her joints, straining under her weight, would be struggling to cope and the resulting damage would eventually develop into early onset arthritis.

Did I miss my chance to make a difference? Have I been a shit GP again? Are doctors slightly egotistical even to consider that a few well-placed words of advice from us can breach deeply entrenched lifestyle and dietary habits? 'Hold on, kids, no more sugary drinks and turkey twizzlers for us. Dr Daniels thinks we are overweight and thank goodness he pointed it out or we would never have noticed. He's given me a wonderful recipe for an organic celery and sunflower seed bake and we're swimming the Channel at the weekend.'

Saving lives

A few years back I spent a stint working in a hospital in Mozambique. Each morning the American consultant would start the ward round with a prayer and then shout boldly and, with not the slightest hint of irony, 'Come on team, let's go save some lives!' The rest of us would then cringe internally, roll our eyes at each other and then follow him round the morning's array of sick and dying Africans. There are a surprising number of Western doctors filing around the wards of African hospitals. I'm not always sure of the motives but there we were: an American cardiologist, two British GPs and a French nurse. Between us, we had years of expensive medical training and lots of letters after our names. As we wandered through the wards, we didn't really save many lives. The majority of our patients were dying of AIDS-related illnesses or malaria. There were no anti-AIDS drugs (antiretrovirals, ARVs) and even our malaria medication supply was low because of a robbery at the hospital pharmacy (an inside job).

Meanwhile, 30 miles outside of town, Rachel, a 22-year-old from Glasgow with no letters after her name, really was saving lives. Rachel had dropped out of her sociology degree and had been working in a call centre before deciding to come and do some voluntary work in Mozambique. She had raised some sponsorship from back home and was touring the rural villages with a troop of local women. All she had at her disposal was a basketful of free condoms and a few hundred subsidised mosquito nets. Accompanied by information and education in the form of songs and posters, her campaign was a raging success. She later e-mailed me to say that malaria deaths had reduced and that she was hoping to have an equally good result with HIV transmission rates.

At the same time, my learned colleagues and I made clever diagnoses on the ward and skilfully inserted chest drains and spinal needles. Occasionally, we did save a life and it was quite exciting when a patient got up and went home after being at death's door. As we waved them off, we knew that ultimately they would be back. They couldn't afford to pay for the full course of medication, and it was only a matter of time before they were unwell again and back in our hospital. We were briefly prolonging lives rather than saving them.

Regardless of the country it is practised in, most of hospital medicine is painting over the cracks rather than fixing the wall. Lives are saved by preventing illness rather than curing it. If you are 64 and admitted to hospital in the UK with a heart attack, it will be all blue lights and running around. After emergency heart scans, a dashing young doctor will probably give you a whack of clot-busting medicine into your veins and it could save your life. At age 16, this was just the kind of exciting medicine that I imagined my job would be. I have been that doctor and at times it is genuinely quite glamorous and exhilarating. Sometimes, it does make a real difference and lives are saved. The patient and family will thank you and you'll feel pretty good for a bit.

Since I have been a GP, on balance I have probably saved far more lives than I did during my time as a hospital doctor. It is my job to try to prevent you from having a heart attack rather than save your life immediately after you've had one. It is far less glitzy and dramatic, but by helping patients control their blood pressure, give up smoking and reduce their cholesterol, I have probably helped prevent or at least delay many hundreds of heart attacks. This might sound like a pathetic attempt to try to elevate GPs and combat an inferiority complex put upon us by years of derogatory comments from our hospital colleagues, but I genuinely think it is true. In the same light, the pressure groups who pushed for the government bill for the smoking ban in public places or who pressed for the introduction of the compulsory wearing of seat belts will have saved more lives than all of us put together.

Public health doctors are those who rather than treating individual patients, look at the bigger picture of health trends across the country and the potential interventions that could help. The rest of the medical profession sneer at public health doctors even more than they do at GPs, but the conclusions of public health doctors influence big decisions made in Parliament and can save and improve many lives. The problem faced by public health campaigns in the UK is the tendency for people to react to being told what to do. In Mozambique, Rachel wasn't faced with angry villagers demanding the 'choice' not to be given free condoms or complaining about the 'nanny state' forcing them to sleep under mosquito nets. Getting the balance in the UK is difficult. The opposition to wearing seat belts 30 years ago and the smoking ban more recently was huge. Our role as GPs is trying to tread the fine balance between giving useful advice and encouragement to make good lifestyle choices whilst not being too paternalistic and patronising.

Kirsty, the trannie

Kirsty had once been a married man with three children, but over the last five years she had spent many thousands of pounds having surgery to become a woman. She had her chin made less square, breast implants and, most importantly, her male organs surgically transformed into female organs. (In post-op trannie circles this is known as having your 'chin, tits and bits' done.) As well as the surgery, there was the electrolysis and oestrogen tablets, not to mention the huge amounts of money spent on boutique clothes, expensive make-up and a Gucci handbag that my wife would die for. The only problem was that Kirsty still looked overwhelmingly like a man. She was six foot two and had broad shoulders and stocky legs. Her 1980s perm and size-eleven feet squeezed into a pair of size-nine stilettos didn't help. Kirsty looked like a rugby bloke who had been badly dressed up as a woman by his mates on a stag do.

'How do I look, Dr Daniels?' Kirsty asked as she flicked her hair and fluttered her fake eyelashes in the worst attempt to be flirty that I've ever seen. 'I've had my boobs redone again. Do you want to have a look?'

'No, no, that's erm fine . . . I'm erm sure that they did a good job.' Kirsty is such a regular at the surgery that she no longer feels the need to have a medical problem to present. She is quite happy to pitch up for a chat and a gossip. She always has a story to tell and is a nice break from the dreariness of afternoon surgery.

For those of you who are interested, the operation is called 'male to female gender reassignment surgery'. There are various techniques but the most popular appears to be cutting off the testicles and inverting the penis. The penile and scrotal skin are combined and used to line the wall of the new vagina and to make the labia. The surgeon makes a clitoris using the part of the penis with the nerve and blood supply still intact. According to the surgeon's website, this enables some patients to orgasm. I haven't yet asked Kirsty about this but I'm sure she would happily tell me all about it given half a chance.

Despite the extrovert exterior, there was a real sadness about Kirsty. The sacrifices that she had made to change her gender were extraordinary. She gave up her marriage and children (only one of whom still talks to her). She lost her job and many of her friends and the pain she describes of the surgery and recovery period is unimaginable. Kirsty now lives slightly on the fringes of society. She is stared at in the street and struggles to find acceptance at every corner. It seems amazing to me that she would have put herself through this much to make the change.

Kirsty, however, has absolutely no regrets. She told me that five years earlier she felt that her only choices were to have the operation or commit suicide. In the nicest possible way, Kirsty is a bit of a drama queen but I genuinely think she means this and the doctors at the practice who knew her as a man agree that she was pretty close to ending her life back then.

Empathy is defined as an 'identification with and understanding of another's situation, feelings and motives'. I like Kirsty but I can't really empathise with her, as I just find it so hard to imagine what it would be like to be so unhappy with the gender I was born with.

Kirsty is quite astute and I think that she has spotted this in me. As she left, she said, 'It's fucking hard being me, you know. You should try being a trannie for a day.'

I did once lose a bet at medical school and had to spend an evening out dressed as Smurfette. I'm not sure it really corresponds to empathising with the emotional and physical turmoil experienced by a transsexual; however, being painted completely blue and wearing a dress and blonde pigtails, it did take me a hell of a long time to get served at the bar.

'It's my boobs, Doc'

Stacy was in her late thirties but the years of smoking and sunbeds made her look much older. She stormed in and sat down with the look of someone who wasn't going to leave until she got what she wanted. 'It's my boobs, Doc.' I must have had a slightly puzzled look on my face, so in order to enlighten me she lifted her top to reveal her large and extremely distorted breasts. They looked like two oval-shaped melons surrounded by a layer of puckered skin and had two nipples drooping off the ends. They were pointing at awkward angles and looked completely disconnected from the rest of her body.

'Something needs to be done,' she demanded. 'I 'ad 'em done ten years ago but they need redoing.'

It turned out that the original surgeon was happy to 'redo' them and his letter from 1998 did clearly state that her breasts would need repeat surgery after ten years. The problem was that he was charging 10K for the redo and, according to Stacy, she didn't have that sort of money. 'I need 'em done on the NHS, don't I?'

My sympathy for Stacy was limited. Yes, she did have hideously deformed bosoms but the local breast surgeons were rather busy removing cancers. I didn't really feel that she should qualify for NHS treatment. I began to try to explain that I wouldn't be referring her today when Stacy began rummaging through her bag, eventually emerging triumphantly with a copy of a women's magazine. She opened it up to a double-spread headlined: 'My Fake Boobs Burst and Nearly Killed Me'. I read on to see that, like Stacy, this woman had had a breast augmentation in the 1990s, but ten years later her implants ruptured and left her in intensive care with blood poisoning.

The prospect of Stacy being poisoned by her exploding fake breasts might have entertained a lesser doctor than me, but then Stacy pointed out the part of the article showing that the poisoned implant lady was taking her GP to court for not referring her earlier. I could see in Stacy's eyes that nothing would give her more pleasure than suing my arse for every penny she could. Defeated and broken, I made an apologetic referral to the surgeons as Stacy looked on smugly.

Two weeks later Stacy stormed back in with the letter from the surgeons stating that she didn't qualify for the operation because of 'PCT funding guidelines'. It was the perfect scenario for me. I didn't really want NHS money spent on Stacy's new boob job but could now blame some faceless managers for it not being done. I was off the hook and happily faked sympathetic noises as Stacy complained about how unfair the world was. A month later Stacy found the money to get her breasts redone privately.

Mr Hogden

I was spending a few weeks working in a very pleasant rural practice. It was nice to have a break from the poverty-fuelled social problems of the inner cities. I had dug out a few ties that I had long since stopped wearing and also rediscovered my best posh accent that I had last used for my medical school interview in 1996. Surrounding the surgery was a collection of very pleasant villages with big houses and twee thatched cottages. It was fox-hunting and green welly territory. During a sweltering few weeks in July, it was a pleasure to be cruising around the countryside doing my home visits rather than stuck in city traffic jams cursing the lack of air conditioning in my car.

Driving down a small country lane, I came across a row of small run-down bungalows. They looked a little out of place in contrast to the rest of the local housing. They were the area's small quota of council housing that the rest of the village tried to ignore.

The patient I was visiting was called Mr Hogden. He lived quietly with his sister in one of the less well-kept bungalows. He was only in his early forties but hadn't left his bungalow for nine years. The medical notes seemed to suggest that this was due to a history of agoraphobia, but more obvious on meeting him was that there would be no way Mr Hogden would have fitted through the door. He was fucking enormous.

Mr Hogden resided in the smallest room of the bungalow. It was about the size of a double bed and was taken up entirely by Mr Hogden himself sprawled out on the floor. He had long since broken his bed and now spent his time on a very old, filthy-looking mattress on the floor. Each of his limbs was made up of several huge rolls of fat with a hand or foot poking out at the end. His head emerged out of a humungous mass of lard that was his torso.

The sight of Mr Hogden sprawled out on the floor was a bit of a surprise but it was the smell that I really struggled with. The bungalow was like an oven in this hot July sunshine and there was only a tiny window in the room that barely let in any air or light. Flies were buzzing around in their hundreds and as my eyes slowly adjusted to the dimly lit room, it became apparent where they were coming from. Unfortunately for Mr Hogden, the flies had found that the warm sweaty crevices between his rolls of fat were a perfect place to lay their eggs. Emerging from his legs and body was a legion of maggots. The sight of the maggots and the horrendous smell were almost too much for me and despite priding myself on a strong stomach I had to do my utmost not to vomit.

'You've got to help me, Doctor,' Mr Hogden pleaded with me as he watched me take in the horror of his predicament. Despite the terrible state in which he was living, this was the first time that Mr Hogden had called out a doctor in the last ten years. He had managed to get to the toilet and back up until now and he simply spent the rest of his time lying on his mattress watching a tiny television that was mounted on the wall of his bedroom. His sister brought him his meals and Mr Hogden had quietly grown enormous without bothering a soul. Until now that was. This was yet another of those moments where I felt completely useless and, like all good cowards, I fled. To be fair, what was I going to do? I could have crouched down and picked the maggots out of Mr Hogden's groin creases but I would have vomited. The flies would have fed off the regurgitated contents of my stomach, only adding to his problems.

I called the district nurses. I felt bad. I did. Really. No, I did. I warned them what to expect and when I bumped into them a few days later, they were amazingly stoical about the whole clean-up operation. They put me to shame. I went back to see Mr Hogden the next week. The maggots were gone but he was still lying on the floor of his squalid little room. We had a chat and talked about how we were going to sort things out. His expectations were low. All he really wanted was to be able to spend his days sitting in the lounge on a sofa and watching the television like a normal person. He was too heavy for the current sofa – hence the filthy mattress on his bedroom floor.

I was feeling guilty about my near-vomiting experience during our first meeting so decided to make it my mission to get him a new sofa. I phoned round endlessly and eventually social services agreed to supply a specially reinforced sofa for the bungalow. I had absolved myself. A few weeks after the sofa arrived I received a phone call from a hysterical Mr Hogden. 'Please, Doctor, come round, please.' Worried that the maggots were back, I avoided lunch and headed over. Mr Hogden was sitting on his brand-new sofa and had been there since it had arrived. Unfortunately, the effect of now sitting upright meant that his huge weight was now all being placed on to one pressure point on his bottom. He had not moved from his sofa since it had arrived and had developed unpleasant pressure sores on his bottom. The material of the sofa had gradually begun to stick to the infected sores and Mr Hogden was phoning me to tell me that he was now completely stuck to the sofa and couldn't move at all.

I couldn't quite comprehend what he was telling me over the

phone, but as I arrived I saw that he was quite right. The material of the sofa and the sores on his bottom had become one. It was impossible to see where Mr Hogden ended and the sofa began. It was not a pretty sight and he had the same pleading look in his eyes that I had witnessed during the maggot incident. He was in a great deal of pain and I was feeling helpless again. I couldn't believe that he had let his sores get so bad without calling anyone. He really needed to go into hospital but this was easier said than done. The first job was to cut him out of the sofa, which required a fair bit of teamwork, a set of garden shears and a very strong stomach. The next task was the more difficult job of physically getting Mr Hogden to hospital. I had ordered a specially reinforced ambulance with a strengthened trolley but, unfortunately, despite best efforts, Mr Hogden just couldn't be fitted through the door. Four paramedics, a nurse, a medical student (I had to bring him along to show him that general practice wasn't boring), several of Mr Hogden's neighbours and I all tried to find different angles or ideas to get him out of the bungalow. In the end the fire brigade had to be called to cut out a wider door. They were reluctant and made Mr Hogden sign a disclaimer promising that he wouldn't try to sue them for damaging his bungalow. Eventually, we got Mr Hogden to hospital. The next day my placement ended and I've no idea what happened to him. I hope he's lost some weight and perhaps gained some quality of life.

Small talk

Drew was a very good-looking guy. He was in his early twenties with big muscles, perfectly chiselled features, blonde hair, blue eyes and a probably fake but nonetheless healthy-looking tan.

'I've got a painful testicle, Doctor. Wondered if you'd have a look at it.'

I was the only male doctor to have worked at this practice for over a year and my first few days were spent seeing a queue of relieved men worried about their genitalia. Some had been worried about their 'bits' for months but had been too embarrassed to expose themselves to one of the female doctors.

So there I was, gently rolling Drew's testes between my fingers, looking for lumps. It can be a slightly uncomfortable situation for the patient in every sense of the word, so I decided to try to make a bit of small talk to put him at ease.

'So Drew, what do you do for a living?'

'I'm a film actor.'

'I thought you looked familiar. Have you been in anything I might have seen?'

'That depends, Dr Daniels, I only really do gay porn.'

'Ah, probably not then, no. You . . . erm . . . must have one of those familiar-looking faces I guess. Definitely wouldn't have seen you in a film. Nothing against porn or anything, except the degradation of women and all that . . . well, not many women in your films, I should imagine . . ?'

There was now only one person in the room who was uncomfortable and it wasn't Drew. I really should remember to limit my small talk topics to the weather and city centre parking problems.

Notes

It is always drummed into us how important it is for us to keep clear, coherent and detailed medical notes. These are apparently real extracts from medical notes. They have been doing the rounds as an e-mail.

1. She has no rigours or shaking chills, but her husband states she was very hot in bed last night.
2. Patient has chest pain if she lies on her left side for over a year.
3. On the second day the knee was better, and on the third day it disappeared.
4. The patient is tearful and crying constantly. She also appears to be depressed.
5. The patient has been depressed since she began seeing me in 1993.
6. Discharge status: alive but without my permission.
7. Healthy-appearing decrepit 69-year-old male, mentally alert but forgetful.
8. The patient refused autopsy.
9. The patient has no previous history of suicides.
10. Patient has left white blood cells at another hospital.
11. Patient's medical history has been remarkably insignificant with only a 40-pound weight gain in the past three days.

12. Patient had waffles for breakfast and anorexia for lunch.

13. She is numb from her toes down.

14. While in ER, she was examined, X-rated and sent home.

15. The skin was moist and dry.

16. Occasional, constant infrequent headaches.

17. Patient was alert and unresponsive.

18. Rectal examination revealed a normal-sized thyroid. (*Thyroid gland is in the neck!*)

19. She stated that she had been constipated for most of her life, until she got a divorce.

20. I saw your patient today, who is still under our car for physical therapy.

21. Both breasts are equal and reactive to light and accommodation.

22. Examination of genitalia reveals that he is circus-sized.

23. The lab test indicated abnormal lover function.

24. The patient was to have a bowel resection. However, he took a job as a stockbroker instead.

25. Skin: somewhat pale but present.

26. The pelvic examination will be done later on the floor.

27. Patient was seen in consultation by Dr Blank, who felt we should sit on the abdomen and I agree.

28. Large brown stool ambulating in the hall.

29. Patient has two teenage children, but no other abnormalities.

30. The patient experienced sudden onset of severe shortness of breath at home while having sex, which gradually deteriorated in the emergency room.

31. By the time he was admitted, his rapid heart had stopped, and he was feeling better.

32. Patient was released to out patient department without dressing.

33. She slipped on the ice and apparently her legs went in separate directions in early December.

34. The baby was delivered, the cord clamped and cut, and handed to the paediatrician, who breathed and cried immediately.
35. When she fainted, her eyes rolled around the room.

Lists

Please don't bring a list of problems when you see your GP. I understand that you might not get to the surgery very often. Perhaps you have to sweat blood to get an appointment. Maybe you had to plead with your boss for the morning off and then beg our receptionist to squeeze you in. In fact, it is probably so difficult for you to get an appointment with your doctor, you've saved up all your niggling health queries that have been building up for the last few months and thought it would be better to get them all sorted out in one visit. Please don't!

We have ten minutes per appointment. That isn't very long, but we GPs pride ourselves in dealing with even quite complex problems during that short period of time. We have to get you in from the waiting room, say hello, listen to your concerns, take a history, examine you, discuss options, formulate a plan, write up your notes and complete any necessary prescriptions or referrals . . . all in just ten minutes! It's amazing that we ever run to time. However, if you have saved up four problems to sort out, then that leaves just 2.5 minutes per problem. That isn't very long and we'll either spend 40 minutes with you and annoy the rest of the morning's patients by running very late, or we'll only half-heartedly deal with each problem and probably miss something important.

This is clearly bad for your health and our indemnity insurance premiums.

If you do have a list of several problems, please warn us from the start and tell us what they all are. I've frequently had patients tell me that they are here to talk about their athlete's foot and then after a leisurely ten minutes casually mention their chest pains, dizzy spells and depression on the way out of the door. If you have got several problems you want addressing, try booking a double appointment or decide what problem needs to be dealt with that day and book in another time for the others. Moan over. Ta.

Ten minutes

I see the ten-minute appointment as the patient's time to use as they so wish. Most patients will fulfil the time in the conventional way with a discussion of a health problem that we then try to collectively resolve. However, any GP will tell you that not all consultations run like this. For example, one of my patients uses the time to tell me about the damp problem in her spare room and another about the affair that she is having with her boss that nobody else knows about. I have one patient who comes into my room, sits down and strokes a toy rabbit in complete silence. Initially, I desperately tried to engage her in conversation, but I have long since given up and now I get on with some paper-work, catch up with my e-mails and check the cricket score on-line. When her ten minutes are up, she gets up and leaves. She doesn't even need prompting, a perfect patient!

Some people would consider these patients time-wasters but I don't have any reason to judge a person's motives for coming to see me. I'm not working in casualty. You don't have to have an accident or emergency to see me. I'm a GP, which basically makes me the arse end of the NHS. If you turn up on time and leave after ten minutes, I'll let you talk about anything. In fact, the three above-mentioned patients are among my favourites. My patient with the damp trouble

97

has been updating me on her ongoing problem for months now. She enters my room agitated and upset and then erupts into a monologue on the woes of damp and the turmoil it is causing her. I do very little during the entire consultation other than pretend to look interested and reassure her that it is all going to be just fine. I do gently point out to her when her ten minutes are up or she would stay all afternoon. She is always eternally grateful that I have listened to her and insists that I have made her feel much better. She then happily goes to the desk to book herself in to see me at the same time next week. I also now know the difference between rising damp, penetrating damp, internal damp and condensation!

As for my patient who is having an affair with her boss, I always enjoy her visits. She is a solicitor's secretary in her early twenties and has been shagging the much older married solicitor for some time. Each visit I get the latest instalment in graphic detail and I am left with an *EastEnders*-type cliffhanger to keep me in suspense until the following week. During the last visit she told me she was pregnant. The solicitor offered her £5,000 to have an abortion but she really loves him and wants his child. What was she going to do? Ten minutes come to an end – cue *EastEnders* closing music: *dum . . . dum . . . dumdumdum . . .* Okay, so yet again not exactly a great use of my expensive training and broad medical knowledge, but I like the intrigue.

I am not completely anal about only spending ten minutes with each patient. Some things take more than ten minutes to sort out and if it is urgent and important then I'll just have to run late. Last week I saw a young woman who had been sexually assaulted by her uncle. She wanted to talk to someone about it and for some reason she chose me. I listened for nearly an hour because that is how much time she needed. My subsequent patients were annoyed by my lateness, but she was by far the most important patient I had seen all week and the sore ears and snotty kids had to wait.

Alf

It's a Sunday and I'm working a locum shift in A&E to make a bit of extra money. I used to work in A&E during my hospital training and quite like going back to work the odd shift. It helps keep me up to date with my A&E skills and also makes me happy that I'm not a full-time A&E doctor any more. I pick up the notes for my first patient of the shift, open the curtains and lying on a trolley in front of me is Alf.

'Oh bloody 'ell. Not you. You're bleedin' everywhere, you are.'

Although these were Alf's words, they also very closely reflected my own thoughts.

I had been visiting Alf at home all week as his GP and then I turn up for a shift in A&E to get a bit of excitement and escape from the daily drudge of general practice . . . and there is Alf lying in front of me.

Alf is in his late eighties and lives alone in a small run-down house that he can't really look after. Alf's notes state that he has had 23 A&E admissions in the last five years, which qualifies him to reach the status of 'frequent flyer' in A&E talk. If hospital admissions could earn you loyalty points, Alf would be able to cash his in for two weeks of dialysis and a free boob job. Unfortunately, all Alf's hospital admissions have actually earned him is a bout of

MRSA and a collective groan of disappointment from the A&E staff when they see him being wheeled into the department.

Given the large amount of time Alf spends coming in and out of hospital, you would think that he had a huge list of complex medical problems but, in fact, Alf doesn't really have much wrong with him physically. His admissions have been almost purely 'social'. This means that Alf is admitted to hospital costing a large amount in time, resources and money, because he can't really look after himself at home. When they talk about bed crises and patients on trolleys in corridors, it is because patients like Alf are lying in hospital beds that they don't really need.

This is what happened to Alf this week. I got a phone call from his worried neighbour on Monday saying she had heard him shouting through the wall. I couldn't get into the house so I had to call the police to break the door down. Once inside we picked up Alf, who was basically fine but had fallen over as he often does. Sometimes there are specific reasons why elderly people fall over such as blood pressure problems or irregular heart rhythms. Sometimes elderly people just fall over because they are frail and have poor balance. Alf falls because he refuses to use his three-wheeled Zimmer frame ('it makes him feel old'), because his house is filled with clutter that he refuses to allow to be tidied away and, finally, because he is still rather partial to a large scotch after lunch.

On the Monday I gave Alf a check-over and he was fine. He hadn't bumped his head or broken his hip and insisted that we all 'bugger off' and leave him in peace. Alf looked terrible. He was thin and bony with filthy clothes, long straggly grey hair and quite frankly in need of a good wash.

'How do you feel you're getting on at home, Alf?'

'Fine, now piss off and leave me alone. The race starts in 20 minutes.'

'What about if I got you some help around the house? Perhaps someone to clean up a bit and maybe give you a hand getting washed and dressed in the mornings?'

'I've been looking after myself perfectly well for 70-odd years, I don't need you lot interfering.'

'How about just some meals on wheels to get some meat on those bones?'

'I'm a very good cook, thank you very much.'

Alf had been offered support at home numerous times before, but he had always declined. He was a grown-up and knew his own mind. He sometimes forgot things but he wasn't demented and was entitled to make his own decisions about his own house, health and hygiene. When I got back to the surgery, I phoned social services and asked them to make an assessment. I was specifically going against the wishes of my patient, but Alf was in desperate need of some support and if some nice friendly social worker came and had a chat over a cuppa, perhaps Alf could be persuaded . . . Needless to say the next day the social worker phoned to say that after a brief conversation through the letter box, she had been given the same 'bugger off' as the rest of us.

I can completely see where Alf is coming from. He has lived a long hard life and has managed independently, making his own decisions and doing his own thing. Why should he suddenly have strangers in his house interfering? He wasn't harming anyone other than himself, so why didn't we just leave him alone? I imagine his biggest fear was being carted off to a nursing home and losing his independence completely.

My problem was that as Alf's GP, I had a duty of care for him. That and the fact that his bloody neighbour always called me first when she heard him shouting and swearing through the wall. At least we had a spare key now and so I visited Alf three times that week and each time I picked him up, checked him over and was given the same emphatic 'bugger off' when I offered to bring in some help.

On Sunday morning, the surgery was closed so when Alf fell over, the neighbour just called 999. The paramedics decided to bring in Alf despite his protests and here he was, looking uncomfortable and unhappy on the trolley in front of me. As ever, I checked him over and, being in A&E, I had the advantage of being able to get a quick ECG (electrocardiograph – heart scan) and urine sample checked. They were both normal and predictably Alf just wanted to go home. The problem was that there was no hospital transport on a Sunday to take him home. The ambulance crew wasn't allowed to take him and he didn't have any money for a taxi. We had no choice: Alf had to be admitted to a hospital bed. As he was being admitted to a medical ward, he was subjected to the obligatory blood tests and chest X-ray. Then he would be assessed by the physios and the occupational therapists who would each in turn be told to 'bugger off', until eventually Alf would be sent home only to fall over a few days later and hence the cycle would be repeated.

The government in its wisdom has worked out that patients like Alf are costing an absolute fortune because he is part of the 10 per cent of frequent flyers who are responsible for 90 per cent of hospital admissions. The problem is that it is very difficult to keep patients like Alf out of hospital. Even elderly people who do accept help still fall over or become confused when they get a simple infection. Carers, neighbours and relatives do their best but they don't have medical training and when faced with an old person on the floor, they often call an ambulance. I don't have an answer for what to do with patients like Alf. Perhaps smaller cheaper community hospitals or specially adapted nursing homes that offer short-term care would be a better option. It is such a shame that A&E departments full of well-trained staff and expensive equipment are seeing their beds filled up with social admissions like Alf rather than the accidents and emergencies that they are intended for.

Meningitis

Every six months or so, a newspaper will print an article with a headline something like: 'GP MENINGITIS BLUNDER – My GP diagnosed my child as having a cold, ten hours later she was in intensive care with meningitis.' This is the sort of story that terrifies every parent and every doctor. For GPs who are also parents, it is a double-fear whammy.

Meningitis is a frightening condition for GPs because it tends to affect children and young people and if we miss it, the patient can be dead within hours. The difficult truth behind the scaremongering headlines is that any child who is seen by their GP in the first few hours of meningitis will probably be sent home with some paracetamol having been told that they have a viral infection. Early meningitis symptoms are generally a fever, feeling a bit lethargic and not being very well. We see bucket loads of children like this every week. The symptoms of a rash and neck stiffness that give away the diagnosis are only seen much later on, by which time the child is already quite sick.

I know an excellent and experienced GP who sent home a child who then went on to develop meningitis. It is a horrible diagnosis to miss but only rarely is it a 'blunder'. The only thing we GPs can really do for the thousands of snotty feverish children we see every day is educate the parents as to what danger signs to look out for and when to bring them back to see us.

I've only seen meningitis a handful of times and thank goodness never as a GP. The first time I saw it was the most memorable. I was working in casualty and a dad carried his four-year-old child into the waiting room. I took one glance at the child and went straight to the drugs cupboard, whacked some penicillin into his vein and called the paediatric registrar instantly. Despite the fact that I had never seen meningitis before, the diagnosis was obvious. The child looked really bloody sick. He was floppy and completely disinterested in anything around him. This was not a clever diagnosis. No doctor in the world would have sent this child home. Several hours earlier when the child was just a bit hot and bothered but still happily watching Disney videos and playing with his brother, the diagnosis would have been much more tricky. If I'd seen the child at this stage, I could easily have sent him home and become the next day's 'blunder doctor' newspaper headline.

I am always happy to see children and babies in my surgery and will do my best to fit them into a full surgery if Mum or Dad is worried. In fact, seeing kids is one of my favourite parts of being a GP. The main difference between children and adults is that kids are very rarely unwell. The truth is since I've been a GP, I've probably seen well over a thousand children and babies, but I am yet to see one that was unwell enough for me to be really worried. Meningitis is really scary but also pretty rare. I understand that this might not be that reassuring if it is your own child that is hot and miserable and that is why I'm always happy to see kids and to reassure parents. As a parent myself, I do realise that it is hugely anxiety-provoking to have this small person for whom you are solely responsible and whom you love overwhelmingly and unconditionally. We doctors are equally anxious when our kids are unwell and I once heard of a GP rushing her infant to see an ear, nose and throat specialist as she was convinced her child had a nasal tumour. She was understandably very embarrassed when the specialist then removed an impressively big but definitely benign bogey from her child's nostril.

A few kids need a good check-over before I've reassured myself that they can go home, but the vast majority are obviously fine as soon as they walk through the door. This may seem a bold statement to make when I've previously talked about how easy it is to miss meningitis early on. However, these borderline kids are the minority of children we see. If a child skips into my consulting room and gives me a smile, they haven't got meningitis. I can't say that they won't develop meningitis in 12 hours' time but then I couldn't say that any well child wouldn't develop meningitis in 12 hours' time. Unfortunately, that is the nature of the disease. In the same way that it took me about one second to decide that the child with meningitis was really sick, it takes me about one second to decide that 99 per cent of the children I see are completely fine.

When I say that the vast majority of the children I see are 'fine', I don't mean that they are not unwell. What I mean is that they don't have meningitis or any life-threatening condition that needs hospital admission right then. They also almost certainly don't need antibiotics as they invariably have a viral infection. It's important that I don't use the word 'fine' to Mum and Dad as they have been up half the night with a miserable crying infant. These children are ill but not ill in a way that I can do anything about. It is just part of being a child.

Kids get ill because they haven't been exposed to lots of the bugs that we have. They are going to be snotty for much of their early years and often spend the vast majority of their first couple of winters going from one viral infection to another. Children need to build up their immune systems and, unfortunately, the only way they can do this is to be unwell. I often think that new parents are a bit unprepared for this part of parenthood. Children will have recurrent ear infections, coughs that last for weeks, sore throats that are really sore and funny spotty rashes that don't quite look like anything in my dermatology textbook. All these things are just part of being a kid and staying up all night comforting them is part of being a parent. It's not much fun at the time but it's normal. I would love to be able to give an instant cure for these childhood illnesses but, unfortunately, I can't. My job is simply to listen to the parents, do a quick examination, offer encouragement and reassurance and make sure that Mum and Dad come back if they are worried. A generation or two ago when big extended families lived together, this reassurance was given by Grandmother or Auntie, but nowadays parents can be quite isolated, hence it is often the GP that fills this role.

Soothing anxious parents is definitely one of the hardest parts of my job. Many are very happy with some sensible reassurance. Others are looking for antibiotics and won't be happy unless they leave with them. We all want the best for our child and seeing them unwell is hard to bear. I think some parents feel that they are letting their child down if their snotty and coughing infant doesn't get antibiotics. In direct contrast, as I strive to be a good doctor, I am trying to hold back from giving antibiotics. It can be a difficult battle that can go either way.

To try to swing the encounter in my favour, I have developed a battle plan. The first thing that I do is try to empathise and say how the child definitely does have a very bad infection – be it a cough or ear infection or sore throat, etc. I sympathise about how hard it is for the whole family when a child is up all night coughing and crying, etc. Vital is me then telling the parents what a great job they are doing with regular paracetamol and lots of cuddles. My aim is to make them feel that I am on their side and that I realise how exhausted they are with no sleep and a miserable child.

Then I explain why antibiotics aren't appropriate to treat viruses, but still offer them as an option. If I've done my job well, they say no, but feel that it is their decision. Finally, I make sure that they will come back and see me if they are concerned and tell them about the worrying symptoms of meningitis to look out for.

If I've succeeded, they don't come back, as the parent feels more confident and the natural course of these viruses is that the child gets better. Ideally, they also feel a bit more confident about managing the child at home next time they are poorly. When these consultations go well, they are great. When they go badly, they are a disaster and usually either end up with the child getting an inappropriate prescription for antibiotics or an anxious parent getting very upset and dragging their child to A&E.

Uzma

It's 6.30 p.m. and my last patient has just walked in. I'm running on time and I'm due to meet a few friends for a drink after work. Working in offices, they have been in the pub for ages and have a pint waiting for me. If I can just get through this last patient quickly, whizz through some paperwork, I'll be in the pub by seven.

Uzma comes in. 'I need the repeat of my pill, Doctor.'

Happy days! Contraceptive pill checks are a boring part of general practice but quick and easy. I do a speedy blood pressure reading, ask if there are any problems, which invariably there aren't, and then the patient is out of the door within a few minutes.

Just as I'm generating the prescription, Uzma seems to be welling up. I'm torn now. I am a nice sympathetic doctor. Honest! It's just that I'm tired and drained and I can practically taste my pint. I really don't fancy spending the next half-hour listening to a weeping 16-year-old. I contemplate pretending not to have noticed, but it's too late. The tears have arrived. They are unmistakable, especially as they are now dripping on to my blood pressure machine. I sink into my seat and prepare myself for a long evening.

'So Uzma, you seem a bit upset?' Not exactly reading between the lines, given her quiet sobs have now turned into loud wailing.

'I can't go home tonight, Doctor; they all hate me. Everyone hates me.' More wailing and tears. 'They blame me for everything and always take my brother's side.' Wail wail. 'My parents don't understand me. We've had a massive fight. There's no way I'm going home tonight. No way!'

Uzma's parents are from Pakistan. Perhaps they are forcing her into an arranged marriage or trying to make her drop out of school? I saw a *Tonight* special with Trevor McDonald on this sort of thing. Perhaps I can really help this young woman. I'll need to get social services and the police involved tonight and find her a place of safety.

'Uzma, are your parents very strict with you? Are they trying to make you do things you don't want to do? Do they hit you?'

'Hit me? God no.' Uzma looks at me like I'm an absolute idiot. 'They all just hate me 'cause they're losers. My sister Nadia, yeah. Oh my God, she's such a bitch. Only because she's jealous 'cause she's got a big arse and no boys fancy her and my mum is always moaning at me about doing my homework and she never says nothing to my brother. He does whatever the fuck he likes.' Like the tears, the words are now unstoppable. There are no breaks for punctuation, but only the odd pause to wipe her tears and blow her nose before the next torrent of adolescent anguish is released.

My interest is diminished again. There aren't going to be forced marriages or honour killings. This is just an ordinary 16-year-old having a hissy fit after a row with her parents. Uzma's mum and dad seem fairly liberal all in all. They probably wouldn't be too happy if they knew she was shagging Darren who works in the garage but then that's not a cultural thing, nobody would want their daughter shagging Darren from the garage.

Uzma is still crying her eyes out and is refusing to go home. What the hell am I going to do now? I need some help with this one. I'm rubbish at comforting crying teenagers. Why on earth has this girl come to see me about all this? Surely there must be far better qualified people to deal with this than me. Someone trained in understanding the emotional turmoil of adolescence, someone who finds it rewarding to address teenage angst on a regular basis. Someone with endless patience and empathy and someone who wasn't supposed to be in the pub 20 minutes ago! As she sobs, I do a quick Google search for teenage counsellors in the town. I get a few numbers and phone them but just reach answerphones. They're all in the bloody pub, lucky buggers.

Just as I'm wondering how I'll ever get home, Uzma's phone rings. It is one of those annoying ringtones that is extra loud and the start of an R&B track that I don't recognise because I'm over 20. The tears stop almost instantaneously and she answers the phone, "Old on a minute, Doc. Wassup, Letisha . . . Is it? . . . Is it? . . . Oh my days! . . . Are you chattin' for real! . . . I'm just with the doctor and that . . . I'll be right there.'

The anguish suddenly vanishes. 'Sorry, Doc, I've got to go. My friend Letisha just got dumped. I've got to go round and find out what's going on.'

Before I can say a word, Uzma is gone. Speechless, I sit in silence pondering the mysterious world of the 16-year-old.

Africa

During a holiday in East Africa, I visited some old friends from medical school who were working in a small rural hospital in Kenya. Rob and Sally had been GPs in the Midlands until they decided to sell their house, quit their jobs and commit to three years in Kenya setting up and running a rural hospital.

Rob proudly showed us round. They had been in Kenya for two years and had achieved an enormous amount for the local community. Thanks to their tireless work, there is now an organised maternity unit and a well-equipped medical ward. Rob has also set up an AIDS clinic with free testing and, most importantly, free access to AIDS medication. It is the only one of its kind in the whole region. Rob and Sally have also pushed hard for education and disease prevention and have spearheaded a campaign to encourage mosquito nets. As a result, they have significantly reduced malaria deaths.

Not only had Rob and Sally been working hard treating patients, they have also been single-handedly planning and managing the changes and improvements to the hospital mostly with funds they have raised themselves. My targets in England for the year might be to get a few patients to lose some weight or cut my diazepam prescribing. Rob and Sally's targets were to build a maternity ward and prevent 100 local children from dying of malaria.

Rob asked me to help out with the HIV clinic for the day. There was no appointment system. The patients arrived en masse in the morning and sat patiently outside my room all day until the last one was seen at about 6 p.m. Not a single person complained about waiting and each one thanked me with genuine gratitude and warmth when the consultation finished. It truly was a humbling experience.

My most memorable patient was Cynthia. She had set off from a neighbouring village the night before and, despite being weak with advanced AIDS and TB, she walked the entire 12 miles and spent the night sleeping in the doorway of the hospital along with many other of the morning's patients. She didn't speak any English so a nurse was translating for me. Cynthia was 24 but looked much older. Her two children had both died aged around 18 months and, although never given a diagnosis, they almost certainly died from AIDS-related illnesses. Cynthia's husband, from whom she contracted HIV, left her once she could no longer work and he realised that she wouldn't be able to produce any healthy children for him. Cynthia was alone and her only means of income was digging in the fields. She was still getting up each day and attempting to work, but her AIDS was advanced and she was too weak to dig. The medications for her AIDS and TB were free and were helping, but what she really needed was something decent to eat. 'Where are you going to get your next meal?' I asked via the interpreter. She shrugged her shoulders and then after a long silence looked me in the eye and asked me a question in her native tongue. Waiting for the translation, I assumed that Cynthia would be asking for some money or food. To my surprise, what she actually asked me for was a job. Even in her weak state, Cynthia clearly still felt that she should earn her way and hadn't even considered a hand-out. One of the previous patients had given me six eggs to say thank you for the mosquito net I gave him, so I gave them to

Cynthia and she left with at least some basic sustenance to help her muster the energy for her long walk home.

As an idealistic sixth-former applying for medical school, I imagined spending many long years working in the poorest and neediest parts of the world. The reality is that apart from my brief experience in Kenya, my only other time practising medicine abroad was three short months in a hospital in Mozambique soon after I qualified. The reality of working in an African hospital was really hard. The facilities were limited, the bureaucracy made me want to tear out my hair and the extent of the corruption was terrifying. The experience was incredible and although it was some years ago, I think of that time often and it helps put both my work and life back in the UK into perspective. I'm a more experienced doctor now and could potentially be much more help back in that hospital in Mozambique, but the question is: do I have the motivation to go back?

Rob is a GP with a similar amount of experience to me. The week before we arrived in Mozambique, a woman came to the hospital in the middle of the night in labour with an arm presentation. This means that the baby's arm had been born but the rest of the baby was still inside the womb and basically stuck. Rob, like me, had spent a few weeks on an obstetrics attachment as a medical student but that was pretty much the sum of his experience of delivering babies. Suddenly, as the only doctor around and ten hours from the next nearest hospital, Rob had to do something. The woman needed a Caesarean section, but there simply weren't the facilities at hand. He tried desperately to push the arm back in and deliver the baby but to no avail and the baby died. The mum was extremely weak from loss of blood and exhaustion. The baby needed to be taken out or the mum would die too. Rob cut off the baby's arm and managed to deliver the remainder of the dead baby.

Rob saved that woman's life and I have the utmost respect for him. If he had decided to stay in England, that woman would have undoubtedly died. Throughout this book I've moaned a bit about the fact that I went to medical school to save lives and make a difference but instead I keep lonely old ladies company and dish out sick notes to the work shy. I haven't ruled out the possibility of returning to Africa to practise some genuine 'life-saving' medicine, but right now I'm not sure that I have the emotional strength to hack the arm off a dead baby at three in the morning.

Evidence

I was being dragged round town on a Sunday morning and, despite the fact that I really fancied a coffee and some cake, my wife wanted us to try out one of the new trendy juice bars that had sprung up. The man behind the counter had a silly pointy goatee and a ponytail. I asked him what an acai berry was given that it was going to make up one-fifth of my five berry smoothie. 'It's hand picked from the shores of the Amazon, man.' (I doubted this.) 'It's got 100 times the vitamin C of an orange so a real natural high. You'll be feeling great all morning and it'll keep those colds at bay.' He looked really pleased with himself as he handed me my smoothie and I wondered what other non-sensical medical advice he gave out to his customers. 'Eat a papaya and cure your verruca.' 'Eat some raspberries and your friends will like you more.' I was desperate to tell Mr Goatee Man that there was no evidence to suggest that eating excess vitamin C was of any benefit in keeping colds away and that it wouldn't give me a 'boost', why would it? Added to this was the fact that if I received any more than 200mg of vitamin C, I'd simply shit and piss out the excess so might as well stick to an orange, which was much tastier and cheaper. My wife knows me too well and gave me a look that meant stay quiet and don't embarrass her in public. I took my smoothie and sat down. Irritatingly, it was really nice and made me feel quite revitalised.

Mr Goatee Man and his smoothie are part of a growing trend of advertising and marketing of 'healthy products' with huge claims about medical benefits without any evidence to back them up. This might seem like a typical rant from a closed-minded doctor, but I genuinely have nothing against my patients taking many herbal remedies and dietary supplements. Many of our medicines originate from plants so perhaps some of them may have genuine medical properties. Saint John's wort, for example, is shown in clinical trials to be effective in the treatment of depression. What I object to is health food companies playing on people's fears and anxieties with regard to their health by making unproven medical claims to sell their excessively expensive products.

Doctors work by the rules of something called 'evidence-based medicine'. The principle of this is that if I want to prescribe you something, it should be of proven benefit. In the past doctors gave out all sorts of tonics and pills based on guesswork and trial and error. I'm sure some of these medications were effective and helpful, but many would have been no better than a placebo. Nowadays we are supposed to apply some evidence to everything we prescribe. If you come to see me with high blood pressure, I can think of 10–20 different pills I can start you on. As the patient you need to put your faith in me giving you the most effective pill for your condition. I can make a decision based on my own experiences over the years after having tried a few different pills on a few different patients. Or I can make my decision founded on a trial of over 10,000 people with high blood pressure that looked with minimal bias at which drug or combination of drugs seemed to reduce blood pressure most effectively and with the fewest side effects. These studies are by no means perfect and as an individual you may not respond in the same way that the majority of people did in the study. However, isn't that a more accurate way of deciding your medication than by me choosing which tablet I most like the name of, or which medicine has the prettiest drug rep who takes me out for lunch most often?

Soon after my smoothie, I was stopped in a shopping mall by a guy selling eucalyptus cream for diabetics.

'How does this work?' I ask.

'Well, mate, you know diabetics, yeah? They have bad circulation to their feet and get foot ulcers.' (I can't fault him so far.) 'Well, when you rub this cream into the foot, it improves the blood flow to the skin.'

'Rubbing anything into your feet increases the blood flow.'

'Well, the eucalyptus cream increases oxygen production in the soft tissues.'

'How does it do that?'

'Free radicals and that.'

'Have you got any evidence to show that this works any better than, say, rubbing lard into your feet?'

Mr Eucalyptus Cream Man shows me the back of his jar of cream. It says, 'Formulated specifically with diabetics in mind.'

'That's not really evidence, is it?'

'Is it you who is diabetic?'

'No.'

'Someone in your family?'

'No.'

'Are you going to buy some of this cream, then?'

'Absolutely no.'

'Well, piss off and stop wasting my time. I'm trying to make a living here.'

Really, I'm just as guilty as Mr Eucalyptus Cream Man. Mr Dudd came to see me recently with a bad back. His back aches because, like him, it is 90 years old. The vertebrae are crumbling and his spine has no flexibility any more. He has tried codeine but this makes him constipated and drowsy and I'm reluctant to prescribe him anti-inflammatory tablets because these could give him a stomach ulcer and damage his kidneys. I decide to give him an anti-inflammatory gel to rub on to his back. There isn't really any evidence that this is more effective for back pain than rubbing lard on to his back. I still prescribe it because I don't want to say, 'Sorry, Mr Dudd, your spine is as crumbly as stilton and there is bugger all I can do for you.' Instead, he goes home and every morning Magda his Polish care assistant comes and gently rubs the 'magic' gel into his lower back. Mr Dudd thinks it is wonderful. 'Thank you, Doctor. That gel really helps.' That's the thing about medicines that are shown to be no better than a placebo: they still work because placebos work. As long as the placebo is cheap and doesn't cause any harm, I'm all for them. I am marginally better than Mr Eucalyptus Cream Man because his cream cost £25 and he was targeting vulnerable old people with diabetes who are worried about getting foot ulcers. My ibuprofen gel cost £1.25 and I made an old man very happy (with a bit of help from an attractive Polish care assistant). Interestingly, the cost of the painkilling gels varies between £1.25 and £12.75 depending on the brand, yet all are probably no more effective for back pain than lard, which costs 19p if you buy the no-frills version in Tesco.

Sticking to evidence-based medicine can be very frustrating. For years I had enjoyed advising my patients to drink lots of cranberry juice when they have a urine infection. They always loved this advice. It helped stop the bugs from sticking to the wall of the bladder I used to say. I don't know where I got this information from but it sounded good and someone clever must have told me it at some point. I guess it was just one of those urban myths that we all buy into sometimes. Patients always love a risk-free natural remedy, especially when advised by the doctor.

Unfortunately, a big study recently showed that although drinking cranberry juice can help prevent urine infections, it can't actually rid you of the bacteria once you have an infection. Bugger, sticking to evidence-based medicine can be very boring sometimes.

Carolina

Carolina was 15 and, unlike the vast majority of teenagers who come to see me, she actually spoke to me in normal words and sentences rather than in grunts and shrugs. I had seen her on several occasions with minor problems, but this time she came in wanting to talk about going on the pill. She didn't have a boyfriend but some of her friends were having sex. She didn't feel ready to have sex yet but wanted to make sure that if anything unexpected did happen that she would be protected. She understood all about sexually transmitted infections and knew how important it was to use condoms. She had also looked up online all about the pill and how it worked. I suggested that she spoke to her mum about this but Carolina told me that her mum was a strict Catholic and she couldn't talk to her about sex. We had a long chat and she decided that she was going to take the prescription for the pill away with her and then have a think about things before potentially cashing it in for the tablets themselves. I remember thinking to myself that if I ever have a teenage daughter, I hope she can talk as openly and honestly about sex as Carolina.

A month later I got an angry phone call: 'Dr Daniels, it is Carolina's mother here. I was just wondering if you could tell me the age of consent in this country.'

'It's, erm, 16.'

'In that case, why have I found a prescription for the contraceptive pill under the bed of my 15-year-old daughter? It's got your signature on it.'

It was an awkward moment. My first reaction was to ask what she was thinking looking under her daughter's bed. Surely that must be the first rule of having a teenager. Don't look under their beds, as you'll only find something you don't want to know about! Carolina's mum was furious. It was a shame, really, as she came to see me fairly often herself and we actually got on quite well. She was one of those really grateful patients who always thanked me profusely even when I hadn't really done much. She was Polish and I romanticise that in Poland they have an old-fashioned respect and admiration for their doctors long since vanished in the UK. The problem was that alongside the old-fashioned value of respecting doctors was the old-fashioned value of expecting your teenage daughter to keep her virginity until her wedding night.

The rules on prescribing the pill to minors are fairly clear. Girls under 16 can go on the pill without their parents' permission. They must have capacity, which basically means that they are able to understand the decision they are making and the pros and cons. As the doctor, I am supposed to encourage the girl to speak to her parents but if I think she will have sex anyway it is recommended that the doctor prescribe her the pill. This was contested in 1983 by a Catholic mother called Victoria Gillick. She didn't want her underage daughters being given the pill without her permission. She lost the case. Interestingly, although under-16s can make their own decisions about treatments that they want, they can't refuse treatment. For example, if a 15-year-old has appendicitis and needs to be operated on but she or he declines surgery, the parents can overrule the decision.

For me, prescribing the pill for 15-year-olds is something that I do fairly frequently. Some people feel that as a GP prescribing the pill, I'm encouraging underage sex. As far as I'm concerned, teenagers are influenced by friends, music, TV and magazines. They're not influenced by slightly geeky 30-year-old doctors with bad hair and Marks and Spencer's trousers. She might later regret having her first sexual experience too young, but she'll be more damaged by having an abortion or a baby. The decisions are much harder if the girl is 14 or 13 or if the boyfriend is much older. It is such a grey area. If Carolina had a boyfriend who was 16 or 17, I guess that would be okay. What if he was 20 or 25? When do I break confidentiality and call the police or social services? These sorts of issues are difficult to judge but faced by GPs every day. I imagine that doctors who have strong religious convictions or those who have teenage daughters themselves may view the whole issue very differently from me.

Back to Carolina's angry mum. I was a bit stuck. I wanted to tell her how sensible her daughter was and that the very fact that the prescription hadn't been cashed in demonstrated her maturity. The problem was that I owed Carolina her confidentiality and couldn't really say anything to mum at all other than to explain that I was within the law to prescribe her daughter the pill. I did sympathise with Carolina's mum. Although I remember feeling very grown up at 15, it is pretty young really. I wasn't having sex at 15 but that wasn't by choice. My combination of bad skin, unfashionable clothes and a disabling tendency to blush and then stammer awkward nonsense whenever within about 15 yards of a girl, meant that I didn't lose my virginity until my late teens. Perhaps my opinions will change in the future, but at the moment I sort of feel that at around that age teenagers will want to be having sex. They will probably make mistakes and have experiences they regret, but if my teenage-girl patients can get into their twenties without getting pregnant or becoming riddled with venereal disease, then I'm probably doing a good job.

Lee

Lee was 36 and was just out of prison. He had been due to be my last patient of the morning but his appointment was at 12.20 and he turned up at 1.30, just as I was about to leave the surgery to do a visit and grab some lunch. I was in the office and could hear him getting slightly aggressive with the receptionist as she explained that I wouldn't see him. It was only fair that I went out and gave her some support.

'Are you the doctor? Will you just see me quickly? I need something to calm me down.'

'No, you're over an hour late so you'll have to rebook in to see me or one of the other doctors this afternoon.'

'Well, can you just give me something to help me sleep?'

I'm not a big fan of prescribing sleeping tablets such as diazepam. I try to avoid prescribing them myself, but looking through Lee's medication list on the computer, I saw that he had a repeat prescription of diazepam still on his screen from before he went into prison. The computer showed he had been prescribed diazepam regularly for years and so I agreed to let him have a prescription for a week's worth now with the plan to start cutting them down at his next appointment. I quickly printed and signed his prescription for diazepam and booked him an appointment for later that afternoon.

That was my one and only consultation with Lee. It took place in the reception area of the surgery and I dished him out a few pills to get him out of my hair so I could get on with my day. Lee didn't attend his afternoon appointment and by the next morning he was dead, having taken an overdose the night before. I read and reread the automatic and very impersonal fax that is generated for every A&E presentation:

Dear *Doctor Daniels*,
Your patient was admitted at *03.45* with a presentation of *overdose*. He was discharged with a diagnosis of *death*.

I felt like shit now. Had Lee overdosed on the medication I prescribed him? I hadn't seen Lee because I was hungry and tired from a long morning surgery and didn't want to get held up. Was that a good excuse? If I had seen him properly and listened, maybe I wouldn't have given him the prescription at all. Perhaps he would have told me a few of his worries, felt a bit better and not topped himself. Had I missed a rare chance to make a real difference? I had an unpleasant morning stewing over Lee's death, imagining explaining myself to the judge.

'So Dr Daniels, the deceased came to see you feeling vulnerable and desperate. He had a history of violence and depression. You were his only source of help and what did you do next?'

'I gave him a week's worth of sleeping pills and told him to bugger off, your honour.'

It didn't look good, did it?

Suicide is a difficult case for GPs to deal with. We see depression and self-harm by the truckload but not many patients actually successfully kill themselves. When I was an A&E doctor, the cubicles were full of teenage girls who had taken eight paracetamol after a row with a boyfriend or parent. There were a lot more cries for help than genuine suicide attempts and most of the 'overdoses' were generally dismissed by A&E doctors as time-wasters. When I was working in psychiatry we saw the next step up. These were genuinely depressed people who took big overdoses and really wanted to die at the time. They only very rarely succeeded in causing themselves any real harm and still ended up in an A&E cubicle with the casualty doctors equally reluctant to have to treat them. Only one of my patients successfully committed suicide during my time in psychiatry. He was a nice young lad of 19 who was just recovering from his first episode of schizophrenia. He had just returned from a gap year travelling round Asia and was looking forward to starting university when he became really psychotic and unwell. He was hearing voices and getting very paranoid. He had to be sectioned and admitted to the ward but he started to improve with medication. I was really pleased with his progress and happy that he was ready to be discharged home. He was realising his potential future of daily medication, psychotic relapses and social stigma. He got into his mum's car, took off his seat belt and drove very fast into a wall. It made me appreciate that, actually, if you really do want to die it isn't that difficult.

I felt pretty shitty when that lad died. The consultant took me aside and said that a cardiologist can't expect to stop all his patients from ever having heart attacks, he just has to look after his patients as best he can and try to prevent as many as possible. It's the same being a psychiatrist or GP. You can't expect to save all your patients from suicide. If I had done everything that I could for Lee, it would have been easier to take. It was the fact that I only really gave him a second-rate service that sat with me so uncomfortably.

After stewing all morning, I phoned the local casualty department to try to find out a bit more about what had happened. The

A&E registrar told me that Lee had died of a heroin overdose. Apparently, it was thought to be accidental. 'There's been a dodgy batch of smack going round town. Caused a bit of a junkie cull. We've had a few of them expire over the last few days. Still plenty more where they came from, I suppose.'

I felt a massive wave of relief wash over me. It was heroin that had killed Lee, not the diazepam I had prescribed him. Lee was still dead and I had let him down as his doctor, but I lived to fight another day. Lesson learnt, I hoped.

Hugging

Would you think it was strange if your GP gave you a hug? Probably yes if you were just asking him to look at your athlete's foot. What about if you were upset and needed some human contact?

One of the GPs near me has been suspended for the last two years for allegedly hugging his patients. He worked single-handedly for many years with no apparent problems, but two years ago, shortly after firing his receptionist, she reported him to the General Medical Council for having had 'inappropriate contact' with patients. A letter was sent to all his past and present patients and one or two of them then confessed that they felt he had been slightly inappropriately tactile with them over the years. Interestingly, nobody actually complained, but he was suspended and is still awaiting the conclusion of an investigation. He is an older GP, originally from Italy, and he claims that he was simply comforting upset patients. I've never met the doctor involved but I've met some of his ex-patients and they explained to me that they always assumed he was 'just a bit Italian' and was simply less reserved than us Brits. I have no idea if there is any truth behind the allegations, but it has made me very conscious of how I am with my patients.

I'm not sure whether there was more than meets the eye with

regard to the Italian doctor, but I do think that cultural differences concerning human contact are important. I saw a very cute little three-year-old Italian girl once. She was very snotty and full of cold but basically fine. After reassuring the mum, she said to the little girl: 'Give the nice doctor a kiss for looking after you so nicely.' I was quite surprised. It just isn't something we do here. I also wasn't too pleased to receive a snotty kiss from a virus-ridden three-year-old.

There also seem to be cultural differences between nationalities with regard to women being examined by male doctors. The general rule for women appears to be that they tend to feel awkward about being intimately examined by a young male doctor until they have had a baby. It would seem that the experience of having legs akimbo and ten medical students trying to feel how dilated your cervix is provides an instant cure for ever feeling self-conscious. Eastern European women seem to feel no embarrassment about stripping off in front of the doctor. I saw a young Czech woman who needed her blood pressure taken. She was wearing a thick jumper and I couldn't roll up her sleeve sufficiently to put the cuff round her upper arm. I asked if she could take off her jumper. She whipped it off without a care in the world and I was rather taken aback to find that she had absolutely nothing on underneath. Not even a bra. The Czech woman herself wasn't bothered in the slightest and this was supported by her normal blood pressure reading. I dread to think how high mine had gone! Later that surgery a woman from Hong Kong came in with a lump on her back. She was absolutely horrified when I suggested that I would need to have a look and in the end I had to send her to a female GP.

I am often faced with somebody very upset and in floods of tears in front of me. They may be someone I've just met or perhaps a patient that I've known for some time and have built up a close relationship with. Regardless of this I just wouldn't give them a hug. One of my GP friends says that he puts a consoling hand on the shoulder of his upset patients. He maintains that it is a comforting form of human contact but not too invasive. I just hand them a box of tissues and try to look sympathetic. I can't think of anything more awkward than a patient asking me for a hug. Funnily enough, though, if they told me that they had rectal bleeding, I wouldn't blink an eyelid about sticking my finger up their bum. Just one of those odd quirks of being a doctor, I suppose.

Tough Life Syndrome

I had a call to visit Jackie again. She is in her late thirties and lives in a tiny two up two down council house with her three teenage children. The house is thick with smoke and painfully cramped. The TV takes up most of the lounge and lying on the sofa in front of it was Jackie.

'You've gotta help me, Doctor. It's the pain. I can barely walk. Those pills don't work. None of it works!'

Jackie has been a patient at my surgery for years. She switches from doctor to doctor and has been on almost every painkiller known to modern medicine.

'Are you going to see Jackie?' my colleague asked me as I picked up her notes and headed out of the door of the surgery. 'She's got the worst case of TLS I've ever seen.' TLS stands for 'tough life syndrome'. Jackie has had a really tough life and this now manifests as chronic pain and fatigue. Jackie was abused as a child and young teenager by her stepdad. She then ran away from home and worked as a sex worker for a bit before she became pregnant at 17 by an abusive partner. Two more abusive partners and two more children later, she was alone at 21 with three children and an alcohol problem. Her children are now teenagers. Her son threatens her and regularly steals her benefit money and her daughter is a heroin user. Her eldest son is constantly in and out of prison. It's not exactly *The Waltons*.

Jackie has pain all over her body. Her abdominal and back pains have been fairly constant over the last ten years or so and now she has general pains in her legs, arms, chest and hands. Jackie has had multiple scans and X-rays that have all been normal. She has seen neurologists and rheumatologists who have examined her thoroughly and run specialist blood tests and scans looking for rare disorders. They all drew blanks. She was finally diagnosed last year with fibromyalgia. The definition of fibromyalgia is 'fatigue and widespread pain in the muscles'. It is a diagnosis of exclusion which means that we diagnose it when we haven't found anything else that could be causing the symptoms.

Officially there is no known cause for fibromyalgia, but time after time when I dig deeply in to the sufferer's past, I find stories of trauma, abuse and unhappy childhoods. Perhaps in years to come they will find some odd hormone or virus that is responsible for this condition and find a cure, but in my experience it almost always occurs in people who have had tough and troubled lives and can't articulate that pain verbally so it is expressed instead as physical pain.

I'm clearly not the first doctor to have recognised the likely association between Jackie's physical symptoms and her emotional state. She has been tried on antidepressants and been referred to counsellors in the past, but she has always been reluctant to accept them. 'I'm not depressed, Doctor. If you could just get rid of this pain then I'd be fine.'

Whenever I visit Jackie she wants me to try her on a new painkiller. Giving out a quick prescription is the easiest option for me as it is the quickest way that I can get out of the house. The problem is that I know that whatever I prescribe won't work. She has tried every painkiller I can think of and now the only step up from here is morphine. I really don't want to be responsible for making her a medicalised heroin addict; besides I know her kids will steal it and either take it themselves or sell it on the estate. Perhaps if I could just help her take some ownership of her condition and recognise the psychological element to it, maybe I could genuinely help her.

'Jackie, why do you think you're having all this pain?'

'I dunno. You're the doctor.'

'It looks like you have had quite a hard time over the years.'

'You can say that again.'

'Some people find that going through large amounts of stress and upset can contribute to having physical pains and low energy.'

'You think I'm making it up, don't you? This pain is real, you know.'

'I don't think you're making it up, Jackie. The pain is real but I just think that perhaps all the stress you've been through might be a big component to your symptoms.'

'Nobody believes me. You doctors are all the same. You can't leave me like this. I need something for the pain. I'm only 39 and I've not been out of the house for weeks. That can't be normal, can it? You have to help me. I need something for the pain!'

'I'm sorry, Jackie, but research has shown that fibromyalgia doesn't really respond to painkillers. Some people find that gradually increasing activity levels and exercise can help. I could also refer you for some specialist talking treatment called cognitive behavioural therapy. There have been some studies to suggest that this can be useful.'

'So you're basically doing nothing for me.'

'I'm not sure what more I can do, Jackie. I'm sorry.'

Doctors tend to deal with patients like Jackie badly. By simply organising more tests and giving more drugs we are positively reinforcing the idea of the sufferer having a medical illness that is the responsibility of the medical profession to treat. The years of hospital out-patient appointments and specialist referrals encourages the idea that the person is sick. It is a role that they subconsciously fill and become dependent on. Being labeled as 'ill' is a distraction from the fairly miserable social and emotional problems that are the underlying problem. In some cases being 'ill' is also a way of exerting some control on the people around them.

My best efforts at trying to gently persuade Jackie to start thinking about the connection between her physical and emotional health were clearly spectacularly unsuccessful and the next time she requested a home visit she specifically asked to see any doctor other than me. I know that this means I have failed, but I have to admit that it is a real relief to know that I won't have to stand awkwardly in her lounge feeling helpless as I watch her suffer. One of my colleagues visits her instead and starts her on morphine.

Mrs Briggs

It is 3 a.m. on a Sunday night and I'm working on call for the 'out-of-hours' doctors. I get a call through to do an emergency visit. Before I arrive, I have only minimal information about what to expect. All I know is that I'm visiting Mrs Briggs who is in her seventies and has breast cancer.

When I arrive, five or six family members greet me at the door. I'm ushered upstairs in hushed silence and shown into a dimly lit bedroom. In front of me lies a skeleton of a woman. Pale and semi-conscious, she is quite clearly dying. In my years as a doctor I've seen many people die. In hospital it is all quite clinical. It is easier to think of them as the 'stroke' in bed 3 or the 'lung cancer' in cubicle 2, rather than as a real person. In the patient's own home it is less easy to protect yourself from the enormity of somebody's death. Surrounded by belongings and pictures of them looking healthy and contented during happier times, the dying person feels overwhelmingly real.

The daughter explains to me that her mum's wish is to die at home and the family is determined to keep her out of hospital or hospice. Up until now she had been managing fairly well, drinking small amounts and her pain was well controlled with tablets. Unfortunately, over the course of the evening she had deteriorated quite rapidly and she was now agitated and seemed to be in pain. She was writhing around the bed and crying out. With end stage cancer, it is very unpredictable as to how and when someone will actually die. With heart attacks, it is easy to understand. The heart ceases being supplied with blood and oxygen so it stops and that's it. A slow-growing tumour that spreads and eats you away from the inside makes you weak and frail but it is difficult to know exactly how and when it will finally kill you. I couldn't be sure exactly what it was that was going to end Mrs Briggs's life, but there was no doubt in my mind that she was going to die tonight.

One of the principal aims of palliative care is to keep the patient pain free until the end. Mrs Briggs was only semi-conscious and couldn't answer my questions. I couldn't be sure of exactly how aware she herself was of the pain, but she was certainly agitated and appeared distressed and I couldn't leave her like this. It was also very upsetting for her family and they were desperate for me to do something. Mrs Briggs couldn't take anything orally so I was going to need to give her an injection of something and that something was morphine. Since Harold Shipman, GPs have been extremely nervous about using morphine in this way. Dr Shipman used injections of morphine to kill his patients and so, understandably, my decision to inject a syringe of the stuff into Mrs Briggs wasn't one to be taken lightly, especially as I knew that she could potentially die quite quickly as a result.

In an ideal world I would set up a syringe driver, which is a pump that slowly injects morphine automatically into the patient until the pain is controlled. But it was 3 a.m. and Mrs Briggs needed pain relief now. There was no way that I was going to be able to organise a syringe driver tonight. I took the family aside and explained that I wanted to give her an injection of morphine. I explained that it might decrease her level of consciousness but would ease the pain and agitation. The family was well aware that she only had a few hours left and they wanted them to be peaceful and pain free. They were happy for me to give the injection. I drew up the morphine into my syringe and slowly injected the clear fluid under her skin. In front of my eyes, her tense agitated body relaxed. I only gave her a few mils, but she had so little flesh on her that she didn't need much for it to take effect. As Mrs Briggs's writhing body calmed, so did the torment on the faces of her family. Her breathing became shallow and she slipped into a deep coma and died a few hours later.

Her family was immensely grateful. It wasn't euthanasia, but perhaps my injection of morphine sped up her death by a few hours. Many of my day-to-day actions as a GP lead me to question the ethics of the choices I make. However, I never doubted that my decision to give Mrs Briggs morphine that night was the right thing to do. My fears about giving morphine are more about the family and how they might react. If I had thought that the family wasn't on my side, I wouldn't have given the morphine. Not because the wishes of the family are more important than the wellbeing of the patient, but because I wouldn't want to have to defend my actions in court. Mrs Briggs would have suffered but I'm not prepared to be labelled as the 'next Shipman'. People accuse doctors of playing God by choosing when patients live or die and sometimes we do, but as long as our decisions are made with compassion and not arrogance, I'll make no apologies.

Betty Bale's cat

Betty Bale is the only patient that I can remember from my first six-month stint as a doctor. She was admitted to my ward on my first day and was still in that same bed when I finished six months later. She was only in her late sixties but had suffered a severe stroke, which meant that she was pretty much completely paralysed. She could speak but it was slurred and she dribbled. It was always an effort to make out her words and even more of an effort for her to say them. She couldn't swallow so had to be fed through a tube running straight into her stomach. All in all, it was a fairly miserable existence.

Strokes are unpredictable and some people recover all of their function, others none and most something in between. For the first few weeks, Betty had intensive specialist physio and speech therapist input, but it soon became clear that she wasn't going to recover much of her movement. Previously independent, this was very difficult for Betty to accept. It was sensitively suggested by the consultant that she would need to go to a nursing home to be looked after. Betty's speech was poor but she made it crystal clear where he could stick his nursing home idea. 'I'm going home!' she would shout as best she could. 'I want to see my cat.' Betty's mind was as sharp as ever. She wasn't confused about her diagnosis, she just hadn't accepted it. If her disabilities had been more manageable, she could have gone home with carers visiting regularly. Unfortunately, Betty needed 24-hour nursing care because of her swallowing problems and severe paralysis.

Betty was taking up a hospital bed on an acute medical ward. It was a complete waste of resources as we were doing nothing for her, but she refused point blank to go to a nursing home and so what could we do? With intact marbles, we couldn't ship her out against her will so we were stuck. Each morning we would do our ward round leaving Betty to last. Doctors hate feeling helpless so none of us really wanted to go in to see her. As the most junior member of the team, I was usually thrown in to say hello. My attempt at a friendly 'good morning' was always greeted with a stoical 'I want to go home' and invariably an 'I want to see my cat.' Betty had never married and had no children. She had painfully few visitors and we often heard her crying to herself as we hurried past her room. It was a miserable situation but one that seemed impossible to solve.

It was decided between the junior doctors and nurses that we were going to bring in her cat for a visit. We knew that if the consultant or, worse still, the infection control nurse found out, we would all be for the high jump, but after so many months of feeling so incapable of helping Betty, we decided we were finally going to do something for her. It was agreed we would sneak the cat in on her birthday. Like a military operation, the cat was picked up from Betty's neighbour and smuggled on to the ward. The cat was a miserable old moggy with clumps of missing fur and she hissed at anyone who came close. We couldn't believe that this was the precious creature that had been so desperately missed. Betty was, however, over the moon. 'My cat, my cat!' she cried. The cat herself seemed less than overwhelmed by the reunion but did at least allow Betty to hold her for a few minutes and even seemed to let out the odd token purr.

It would be nice to finish the story with Betty making a miracle recovery because of the amazing healing power of feline friendship, but that didn't happen. Betty was still paralysed and eventually, after many reluctant months, did have to go to a nursing home. Betty's case sticks in my mind because it shows how despite all the wonderful facilities that modern hospitals contain, it was a mangy cat that made one woman's suffering lessen for a short period at least.

Vaccines

Sebastian was three years old and looking fairly miserable. He was very sweet and, despite being a bit unhappy and feverish, he was keen to tell me that he had a stethoscope like mine at home. His mum had brought him in as she was worried about his rash. He was covered in spots. 'Has he had all his jabs?' I asked casually as I took a closer look. 'No, we don't believe in vaccines,' Mum replied matter-of-factly. I was shocked. I had mostly worked as a GP in working-class areas and never come across anyone who didn't vaccinate their children. This day I was working in a leafy north London suburb and discovered it was almost the norm here.

A lot of what we do as doctors is patch people up and keep them going for a few extra years. There is a lot of listening to people's general health grumbles, giving a bit of reassurance and sending them out of the door with a pretty ineffectual tablet. Medicine is better than it was a hundred years ago but the main reason people live longer and only very rarely die in childhood is due to improved sanitation and nutrition. Clean running water and an abundance of food have saved far more lives than doctors and our medicines. Having said that, I believe the one great achievement of modern medicine is the widespread vaccination of children. Vaccines are cheap, safe and have saved millions of lives both here and all over the world. Measles used to be a major killer in the UK and it has now become a disease that I had only ever read about in textbooks. Despite working as a paediatric doctor both in England and Africa, I had never seen a real-life case of measles.

Until this day, that is. Here it was in front of me, the widespread rash all over the body and the classic lesions in the mouth. I 'Googled' measles and, sure enough, Sebastian's rash looked the same as the one on my computer screen. My final test was to grab Sue, our oldest receptionist, and bring her into the room. 'Is this measles?' I asked her. Taken aback but flattered to be asked her medical opinion, Sue took a quick glance and said, 'That's it. All four of my kids have had it.' There it was: measles, a disease that killed millions of children before widespread vaccinations almost eradicated it completely. As a doctor who had only practised medicine in the twenty-first century, I should never have seen this disease. Measles was back and had become a disease of the middle classes. A disease of Hampstead, Wimbledon and Harrogate – so frustratingly unnecessary.

I was actually quite angry. Sebastian's mum was unrepentant. 'I think it is important for my child to build up his own natural immune system. He is on a special whole-food diet that boosts it naturally.' I was fuming now. 'The immune system is very specific,' I tried to explain calmly. 'The only way that Sebastian can become immune to measles is to either have the vaccine or to have the disease itself, assuming he survives it. He can eat all the organic dates and wholemeal rice in the world, it won't give him immunity to measles, mumps, rubella, diphtheria, tetanus, meningitis C, whooping cough, haemophilus influenza and tuberculosis. These really aren't nice illnesses, you know!' It was not the time to be angry as Sebastian was quite unwell. There is no cure for measles but having no experience of the disease, I wanted the paediatricians to check him over. I sent them up to the hospital with strict instructions for Mum to keep Sebastian isolated from the other children in the waiting room.

Not all children can have vaccines. They can be harmful to children who have diseases of their immune system such as HIV or those having chemotherapy for cancer. Previously, these children were protected because healthy children were all vaccinated and so a disease outbreak was prevented. Now that healthy children such as Sebastian are no longer being vaccinated, these vulnerable children are at risk. The last thing a child on chemotherapy needs is a bout of measles. Vaccinating isn't just about protecting your own child.

Darryl

'What can I do for you today, Darryl?'

''Allo Dr Daniels. How are you?'

'Fine, thank you, Darryl.'

'I 'ope you're 'aving a good day and that.'

Darryl was a local thug who had somehow avoided ever having been locked up despite years of fights, assaults and petty crime. He tended to be rude and demanding so his less than impressive attempt at being charming meant that he must have wanted something.

'I need a letter to say I couldn't go to my community service last Thursday.'

'Why was that?'

'I had bad flu.'

It annoys me when people say they have flu when actually they have a bit of a cold. However, it wasn't the time to correct Darryl. He was significantly bigger than me and I have naturally cowardly tendencies.

'Are you still unwell?'

'No, I'm better now.'

'Well, why didn't you come in at the time you were unwell?'

'I phoned up the receptionist and she told me that there were no appointments available except for emergencies. She also told me that my symptoms were probably viral and I should take some paracetamol and go to bed.'

We had clearly trained our receptionists too well and now Darryl had worked out how to get out of his community service without getting in the shit.

'I didn't want to waste an emergency appointment and that.'

How noble of you, Darryl. Such a shame that your high sense of altruistic morals couldn't have been better demonstrated when you were kicking the shit out of some poor lad who'd accidentally spilt your pint. (I thought this rather than said it, for obvious reasons.)

I really didn't want to write a letter for Darryl. I also had had a bit of man flu that Thursday. I had ventured in and spent the day feeling miserable. I didn't see why Darryl couldn't have done the same. I imagine he had a few beers the night before and decided to give the leaf sweeping a miss for the day, knowing he could hoodwink some foolish GP into writing a letter to get him off the hook.

'My probation officer says I need a letter and that. I'm on my last warning for missing community service days. They're threatening to take me back to court and put me away.'

So there I was, writing a letter as if to excuse my child from doing PE at school:

Dear Probation Officer,

We both know Darryl is an unpleasant little scrote who will do anything to slime his way out of trouble and get out of doing any work. He tells me he had a bit of a snuffly nose last week (boo hoo) and now wants me to write a letter so he doesn't have to go back to court to face a breach of his community service order.

Please send him straight to jail and lock him up for ever as I am in a particularly unsympathetic mood due to the fact that I'm running late because of time-wasting twats like Darryl.

Yours sincerely,

Dr Benjamin Daniels

This was the letter I would love to have written. One day I will write it and bask in momentary satisfaction before they suspend me for unprofessional conduct and Darryl comes to my house and beats seven lumps of shit out of me. I hoped the probation officer would read between the lines of the more mundane letter that I actually wrote:

Dear Probation Officer,

Darryl tells me that he couldn't go to his community service last Thursday as he had symptoms of a viral infection. He was not examined at the time and his symptoms have since resolved.

Yours sincerely,

Dr Benjamin Daniels

Nothing in this letter required any small degree of medical knowledge or skill, but the very fact that it was written by a doctor rather than his aunt Doris meant that Darryl would probably get off the hook with the court and avoid going to jail.

The pat dog

My last hospital job before I became a GP was in psychiatry. I already knew that I wanted to be a GP by this stage and, given the large amount of psychiatry in general practice, I thought that it wouldn't be a bad idea to spend six months learning a bit more about mental health. The job I had was actually in forensic psychiatry. I was on a locked ward with patients who were supposedly 'criminally insane'. I loved going to parties and telling people I was a forensic psychiatrist. It sounds good, doesn't it? It gave people the impression that I was akin to the Robbie Coltrane figure in *Cracker*, solving crimes and bringing insane criminals to their knees with my brilliant questioning and diagnoses. The reality, of course, was very different. I wasn't really a forensic psychiatrist, I was the junior doctor attached to the forensic psychiatry team. I wandered around the ward doing the odd blood test and checking blood pressures. Occasionally, I would write a letter to the Home Office asking whether a patient would be allowed to go to his sister's wedding as long as he promised not to drink too much or murder anyone.

The patients themselves were a mixed bunch. They had all committed crimes of some sort while mentally unwell, but many of them didn't really need to be locked away. One of the lads had set fire to a homeless hostel when he was having scary delusions and hallucinations because of schizophrenia. There was no malice involved in his crime. In his psychotic state he had simply been trying to save the other residents by smoking out the evil spirits. His symptoms were well controlled now by medication and he wouldn't have hurt a fly; however, arson is taken seriously so he was locked up on our ward. Another patient became quite paranoid when smoking weed. He got into an argument at a party and stabbed someone. I'm not sure if it was the paranoia to blame or simply the stupidity that lots of young blokes have when a bit drunk and stoned. That was ten years earlier, but he remained on our ward because he was still apparently a danger to society.

Our oddest patient was called Tommy. I'm not quite sure what his diagnosis was but he was on the ward because of his sexual disinhibition. He had never raped or sexually assaulted anyone but he used to expose himself a lot and masturbate in public. Tommy was fairly quiet on the ward and the other patients had learnt to tolerate his odd behaviours. They would quite happily sit in the TV room trying to guess the *Countdown* conundrum while Tommy would be sitting quietly in the corner wanking himself off over Carol Vorderman.

Tommy's behaviours seemed to be getting better with some help from the psychologist and we thought things were going well until the incident with the pat dog. A pat dog is usually a very docile oldish dog that occasionally gets brought round nursing homes and hospital wards. The idea is that spending some time with a friendly dog can make people feel a little better for a bit, maybe even help bring them out of their depression and anxiety. Everyone loves a big cuddly docile dog that likes being stroked.

Trigger was just this type of dog. He was a ten-year-old Labrador who just adored being given attention. His owner was retired and enjoyed bringing him around to the hospital. While Trigger was being petted by the patients, Ted his owner would have a cup of tea and a chat with the nurses. It was a Wednesday afternoon and I was sitting in the nurses' office writing up some notes. Trigger was in the lounge with the patients and Ted was in the office with us talking about his impending hernia operation. Suddenly, we heard barking. 'That's odd,' said Ted, 'Trigger never barks.' We all rushed into the lounge to see a very upset-looking Trigger being chased around the room by a naked Tommy and his erect member. It shouldn't have been funny, but it really was. We never saw Trigger or Ted again, speculating that the poor dog had post-traumatic stress disorder and had probably been retired early on health grounds.

Rina

'How can I help today?'

   'Pain, Doctor.'

'Where is your pain?'

   'Pain all over, Doctor.'

'Everywhere?'

   'Yes, Doctor.'

'Head?'

   'Yes, Doctor.'

'Legs?'

   'Yes, Doctor.'

'Arms, chest, back, toes, ears?'

   'Yes, Doctor. All-over body pain, Doctor.'

Rina is in her forties and from Bangladesh. She has been in England for many years but, unfortunately, she still speaks only minimal English. I've never seen her smile or look anything other than thoroughly miserable. She often comes in bruised and I suspect that she is hit by her husband, although she denies this. Over the years she has presented with numerous pains all over her body and we have never found a medical cause for them. We call it CHAOS, Constant Hurts All Over Syndrome.

   'Medicine to help me, Doctor? Please, thank you.'

Rina comes to the surgery most weeks presenting with some pain or another. I've never found a cause for the pain and suspect it is related to stress and depression. Rather than fob her off with another painkiller, today I decide to do the right thing and try to treat her holistically. I'm going to treat the whole person. Explore her health beliefs and expectations. Do the right thing.

'So, Mrs Miah, why do you think that you have so many pains?'

'Pains all over, Doctor.'

'Yes, but why do you think you are having so many pains?'

Silence.

'We have done lots of tests and they have all been normal. Some people find that when they have pains all over for a long time, it can be connected to stress. What do you think?'

Silence.

'Is there anything else that you'd like to discuss today? Any problems at home?'

More silence.

I think Rina has understood me but she still looks at me blankly. We both sit there in an awkward silence. Me wondering why she can't talk about her emotions; her wondering why I'm not dishing out a prescription and letting her get on her way. The way we view pain and disease is very dependent on culture and our under-standing of illness and its causes. The concept of rationalising pain and physical symptoms with underlying emotional problems is something that my middle-class English patients thrive on. They love to be asked about how their overall health may be affected by their external environment. 'Hmmm, Mrs James, you seem to have had a lot of colds recently. Why do you think that might be?' 'Well, perhaps I have been overdoing it a bit at work recently and I am very worried about Samuel's school entrance exams. Maybe I should go back to working part time. What do you think, Doctor?'

I have no idea what Rina's ideas are about her health and

whether she ever contemplates any possible external cause for her all-over body pain. I'm not sure if it is a cultural barrier or a language one that I'm facing with Rina. Perhaps she does recognise that she is depressed but can't express it to me for whatever reason. If I was working in Bradford or the East End of London, I'm sure there would be specialist services available for someone like Rina – a place with multilingual support and experts in problems faced by Bangladeshi women in the UK. Unfortunately, this town is small and mostly white. Our counsellors are excellent but I fear that they would face the same language and cultural barriers as me. I once started her on an antidepressant but despite careful explanation as to how they should be taken, she just took them once in a while when she had a pain and so, of course, they didn't help.

Rina's daughter is with her today and is happy to interpret for me. The problem is that, although very bright and articulate, she is only 11 and I don't feel it is fair to use her to help translate personal questions about her mother's mental health. Officially, we should use professional interpreters but it is hard work and time consuming. Even if I can establish that Rina has stress and depression, I probably won't change the things that are making her depressed and it is so much easier just to give a prescription for another painkiller and wave her on her way.

Doctors do appreciate the importance of treating people holistically and recognising cultural differences but that appreciation doesn't always help the individual patients in front of me. Sometimes I blame not being holistic on only having ten minutes per consultation, but I could have ten hours with Rina and I'm not sure whether the outcome would be any better. Yet another unsatisfactory consultation and a feeling of short-changing my patient.

Dos and don'ts

Doctors are fairly immune to seeing you naked. Not much will shock or embarrass us, but if we are going to be required to delve into your nether regions, it would be immensely appreciated if you had a bit of a freshen-up first. Men, if you have a problem with your bits, give them a quick wash before coming into my surgery. I personally haven't had a foreskin for years. I find them an oddity at the best of times. I don't want to have to peel back yours to discover a crusty layer of knob cheese. You will see me gag. Women tend to be a lot more considerate and, if requiring a vaginal examination, will make sure all is presentable. I did hear about one woman who, while running late for the doctor, gave herself a quick spray of what she thought was a vaginal deodorant. It wasn't until she saw a puzzled-looking doctor remove a very sparkly-looking speculum from inside her that she realised she had doused herself with glitter spray by mistake.

Don't ask me how I am. That's my question. We both know that you are here to talk about you. I know you are being polite but one of these days I might just answer the question and spend your precious ten minutes ranting about my cat's fungal infection and my annoyance at my neighbour's choice of late-night music.

Don't ever ever ever say, 'What's up, Doc?' It might seem momentarily amusing but it really isn't. It is the equivalent of shouting, 'I don't belieeeve it' to the actor from *One Foot in the Grave*, or shrieking, 'Riiicky!' to the corresponding *EastEnders* actor. We've heard it before and it just gets less and less funny. Some doctors hate being called 'Doc'. I don't really mind. In my football team there are three Bens but I'm the only doctor so I am affectionately called 'Doc'. 'On the 'ead, Doc' has a certain ring to it. At school I was distinguished from the other Bens by being called 'Big Nose', so 'Doc' is a significant improvement.

Please don't ask us medical questions when we're not at work. I was at the barber's and he asked me what I did for a living. I foolishly admitted that I was a doctor and he then proceeded to unbutton his shirt and ask me my opinion about a rash on his chest. We don't want to answer medical questions on our day off and we certainly don't want to examine you unless you are extremely attractive. I can promise you that this barber wasn't! The awkward part of being asked medical questions outside of work is that I might need to ask embarrassing questions. For example, one of my wife's friends asked me why she kept getting urine infections. When I started talking about the possible pH of her vagina and explaining how different sexual positions facilitate the passage of bacteria up the urethra, she looked rather disturbed. She blushed, made her excuses and has barely spoken to me since. My wife accused me of being inappropriate but at least her friend won't ask me medical questions in the pub again. Some things are just best left for the consulting room.

If you're a smoker, just be honest about it. So many smokers come in with awful chest infections and, when I ask them if they smoke, they proudly state, 'No, Doctor.' When I then ask, 'Did you used to smoke?' They say, 'I haven't had a cigarette for two days.' This doesn't make you a non-smoker and certainly doesn't merit any congratulations from me. The fact that you have felt so breathless and unwell that you haven't managed the ten-minute walk to the corner shop to buy your cigs makes you disabled, not an ex-smoker.

It is actually really refreshing when a smoker walks in and says, 'Yes, Doctor, I smoke. I know that it's bad for me but I like smoking and I don't really want to stop.' So many patients make up a lame excuse that they then recite to me: 'I stopped for a few days and that, but then my sister Amy, she was really upset 'cause Kevin, her bloke, done the dirty on her again and I 'ad to comfort her and it was dead stressful and I 'ad to have a couple of cigs to calm me down . . .'

Home births

Sophie is 32 and about to have her first baby. She is not a patient but a friend. Typically of my generation of middle-class women, she focused on herself and her career before considering starting a family. Up until now every aspect of her life has been very effectively managed. She is used to having complete control and we had joked that her wedding last year was run with ruthless efficiency like a military procedure. Sophie is delighted to be pregnant and, like every big event in her life, she has carefully researched everything there is to know about pregnancy and birth. The single most important conclusion she has made is that she doesn't want her birth to have anything to do with the medical profession.

'I'm not ill, you know. I'm having a baby. It is the most natural thing in the world. Why should I go to a bloody hospital?'

Sophie had long since rejected Western medicine in favour of homoeopathy, acupuncture and herbal treatments. She only eats organic food and her near-daily yoga classes keep her fit. She had never really had to consider conventional medical treatments because she had always kept herself so sickeningly healthy. Sophie felt very strongly about having her baby at home with no medical intervention and she was ready to battle for her cause at any opportunity. We met up for a coffee and she was spoiling for a fight. Much to her disappointment, I am not particularly averse to home births. Evidence suggests that if the pregnancy is uncomplicated, a birth at home is just as safe as a birth in hospital and it is certainly a much nicer environment. My personal reservation about births at home is the possibility of me as a GP having anything to do with them. Gone are the days when a GP would happily get out of bed at 3 a.m. to assist with a difficult home delivery. I have only ever delivered a couple of babies. That was some years ago and I had a very experienced midwife watching my every clumsy move. You really wouldn't want me anywhere near the delivery of your child.

Doctors see the births that go wrong. They are clearly the minority but even in this day and age, babies and – even very occasionally mothers – do still die during childbirth. When you see a problematic birth, it tends to stay with you. Given the choice personally, I would probably put up with unfriendly midwives and bad décor and have my baby in hospital. I would want the reassurance that a team of specialists was on hand should things go tits up. Of course, as a bloke I will never have to make the decision so my opinion is fairly irrelevant.

Home birth advocates would say that delivering your baby at home leads to fewer complications as the mother is more relaxed and this reduces the rate of births that go to Caesarean section. Both of my friends who had opted for home births ended up going on to have a Caesarean after being transferred to hospital by ambulance. Rather than pushing towards home births, shouldn't we try to put more effort into building birthing centres or making hospital a nicer environment to give birth in?

My only other comment on home births is that they are something that I remain immensely dispassionate about. The birthing experience is clearly very important for the parents, but middle-class women complaining that hospitals are a bit sterile and unfriendly is not my biggest concern as a GP. Home births are almost solely a concern for the middle classes. As with homoeopathy, organic food and rejecting the MMR jab, they tend to be the choice of healthy, educated and well-adjusted parents. Whether their child is born at home or in hospital, the child will probably be welcomed into a warm, loving, supportive family.

The births that I am concerned about are those from the young, isolated, council-estate mums who are often bringing their children into less savoury environments. I spend a lot of time trying to make sure that these mothers have the support they need and, with the help of social workers, midwives and health visitors, that the child will be safe from potential neglect and abuse. Sophie feels that a bad birth experience, and particularly a Caesarean, can affect the future development and personality of the child. I personally doubt that is true. I feel that far more important is the mother's ability to make an early bond with the child and give that child a stable, nurtured and safe start in life. Postnatal depression is perhaps the biggest contributor to mothers struggling to bond with their children. This can affect women of all classes and ages, but poverty, isolation and being a teenage mum are, in my experience, the biggest risk factors. I personally would rather money was spent providing for these vulnerable mothers than on funding home births.

Michael

It was a drizzly Tuesday morning in November and Michael was my fourth patient complaining of a cough and sore throat. My initial reaction was that I was seeing yet another case of man flu. Young men make such a fuss when they have a bit of a cold. They demand mountains of sympathy and expect you to discuss with them for hours the merits of Lemsip vs Beechams.

Unfortunately, Michael didn't just have man flu. There was something not quite right. He had already had three courses of antibiotics for recent chest infections and was losing weight. On closer inspection, he also had a white furry tongue that was almost certainly oral thrush.

Michael was 33 and a teacher at the local school. He was from Zimbabwe and had moved to England two years ago with his wife and baby daughter. His symptoms suggested a weakened immune system and I had to consider AIDS as a definite possibility. I discussed with Michael doing more blood tests. It is never easy bringing up the subject of HIV but it was important that I asked him directly about it and whether he felt he had ever put himself at risk. I talked to him about doing an HIV test and counselled him fully on what we would do if the result was positive.

Sexual health clinics are much better than GPs at managing

HIV testing and I suggested that he attended our local walk-in centre. Michael looked horrified. Teachers tend to avoid the clap clinic as there is always a good chance that they'll be sitting in the waiting room surrounded by their teenage pupils. Michael denied that he had ever put himself at risk but agreed to talk to his wife and come back the next day for me to do a blood test.

Michael missed his appointment. I wrote a letter and phoned twice but he never got back to me. I had a dilemma. Michael could well be HIV-positive but didn't want an HIV test. He was, of course, completely within his rights to make this decision, but what about his wife and daughter? They could well be HIV-positive, too, and if diagnosed early, could potentially live long healthy lives on antiretroviral medication. I doubted strongly that Michael had spoken to his wife about his suspected diagnosis. The whole family were my patients so I had a duty of care for them all; however, I couldn't break Michael's right to confidentiality.

I was searching for a solution when one found me. Michael's wife brought in their four-year-old daughter Cynthia to see me because of a lump on her neck. I had no idea if this lump was related to being HIV-positive or not, but it was an opportunity that I couldn't miss. I talked with Michael's wife about the many different causes for neck lumps in children, including AIDS, and discussed the option of a referral to the sexual health clinic for HIV testing. I wasn't breaking Michael's confidentiality but my actions did result in all three of them being tested. Unfortunately, the whole family tested HIV-positive with Michael and his daughter already having symptoms of AIDS.

I didn't officially break Michael's confidentiality but in some ways I did break his trust. He hasn't come back to see me since but instead saw one of the other GPs at the practice. Michael and his wife and daughter were now on antiretroviral drugs and doing well. I feel I can ethically defend my actions; however, I do wonder if I would handle things differently next time. What a relief it was when my next young male patient with a cough and sore throat genuinely just had man flu.

Alternative medicine

I view alternative medicine a bit like I view prayer. I believe that both only work if you really have faith in them. They are also similar in the fact that neither can be explained by evidence or science, yet live on after thousands of years. My own personal belief is that both prayer and most alternative medicine practices only work via the placebo effect. However, as a doctor it is important that I put aside my personal reservations and accept that many of my patients believe in non-conventional forms of medicine. Trying to inflict my own scientific beliefs on to my patients just makes them feel defensive and alienated by modern medicine. I want my patients to feel that regardless of our differing views, they can always come and see me to discuss their health.

As a GP, patients often ask me what I think about specific alternative practices. It is important for me to tell them that they are not all the same. It would be rude to compare a chiropractor with a crystal therapist or a fully qualified herbalist with a faith healer. I am usually fairly non-committal on the subject and say, 'If it works for you, then go for it.' I am particularly keen not to put off my more difficult patients from trying alternative medicines, particularly if it means that they might be encouraged to not visit me quite so often.

One of the original founders of psychotherapy talks about the doctor being 'a drug'. This is the idea that regardless of what we diagnose or what medicine we give, simply our spending time with a patient, listening to them and possibly reassuring them is in itself often an effective treatment for many ailments. This form of healing is perhaps being lost in the modern general practice of targets and ever shorter appointments. Regardless of whether they offer homoeopathy, acupuncture or Reiki healing, the alternative practitioners are filling that gap by giving the time and attention that GPs don't have an opportunity to offer.

One gripe I have with alternative practitioners is that they are ultimately private. Somebody is making money out of your illness and having only ever worked for a free at point of access health service, I find that an uncomfortable concept. I am fortunate enough to have never had any problems with my back, but I am fairly sure that if I presented to a private chiropractor, he would examine me and diagnose me with various weaknesses and instabilities and then recommend a set of ten sessions for £50 a pop. I expect a lot of alternative practitioners do similar things. Doctors working in private practice are no better. I had a patient who returned from a skiing trip in Bulgaria. He had had an accident and injured his leg. The doctors did an X-ray to exclude a fracture, which is reasonable enough. They also did an ultrasound scan, a CT scan and prescribed five different medications. All this for a bad bruise! The doctors were playing on the patient's fears of being unwell and fleeced him for a small fortune. Unfortunately, I think that many private doctors play this game and it is a real relief to me that I don't have the temptation of earning more money by prescribing more drugs and ordering more tests.

Most of what I prescribe as a GP is based on evidence and I talked about this earlier in the book. The concept is that I can't just give any medicine for any ailment. For me to use a medicine there has to have been a large non-biased trial that showed that this medicine worked better than a placebo. For some treatments such as homoeopathy these sorts of tests are fairly easy to carry out and most of the evidence would suggest that there is no difference between a homoeopathic treatment and a placebo. For other alternative treatments, conducting these sorts of trials is more difficult but it can be done. For those of you unfamiliar with Reiki, it consists of a specially trained Reiki 'master' laying his or her hands upon the patient and controlling the energy forces that pass through the body. Advocates of Reiki talk about the amazing feeling of a glowing radiance and heat that passes through them during a Reiki healing session. Apparently, an experiment took place where several actors watched a Reiki master perform and then they imitated his healing technique. When the actors impersonated the healer using realistic but completely made up mystical chants and movements, the patients were just as aware of the radiance and heat passing through their bodies and were unable to tell the difference between the work of the Reiki master and the actors.

Now I would be wrong to criticise a profession for healing via the placebo effect as I use placebos all the time for my patients. The important thing to remember is that placebos do work. As I said, I am fairly sure that anti-inflammatory gel is of no more benefit for chronic back pain than rubbing on a placebo gel. This would suggest that it is the process of rubbing the gel on and thinking that it is reducing the pain rather than any pharmacological properties of the gel itself that are working. However, whether you use a placebo gel or the real painkilling gel, the patient feels better than if they have no gel at all. This is how most alternative medicines work. The mind is an immensely powerful tool for healing and is used by conventional doctors and alternative practitioners alike. If we can convince our patients to have belief and faith in our treatments, the results can be astonishing.

My most dramatic witnessing of the healing power of the mind occurred during my time working in Mozambique. A middle-aged woman presented herself to the ward in absolute hysterics. She owed her village witch doctor money that she couldn't afford to pay and he had put a curse on her. The woman was convinced that she would die shortly and was screaming and throwing herself on to the floor and beating the ground. We managed to keep her still for a few minutes to do some basic observations and I have never known someone to have a pulse and blood pressure so high. It was quite possible that she could die from a heart attack simply because of the immense stress her body was under.

The head of medicine was a German professor who was always particularly impatient with the local people's spiritual beliefs and superstitions. 'There is no such thing as witchcraft!' he shouted at the woman as she writhed and screamed on the ground. The woman took no notice and carried on wailing as her blood pressure and heart rate continued to rise to increasingly dangerous levels. One of the local doctors took a very different approach. 'I can break the spell,' he told her authoritatively. He took some magical stones from his pocket (some gravel from the hospital courtyard) and started chanting and throwing his arms around. After several minutes, he dramatically threw the gravel to the feet of the hysterical woman and announced in a booming voice that she was cured. The woman collapsed into an exhausted heap and started to whimper. Her blood pressure and heart rate were normal within a few minutes and she happily headed home to her village. 'If you look convincing enough, these people will believe anything,' the doctor remarked to me after I had looked on in astonishment. He then calmly asked one of the nurses to sweep up the gravel and we carried on with the ward round.

A patient once told me that she had turned to homoeopathy as she didn't feel that she was treated holistically by modern medicine. I felt a little offended by this. The different ways in which health and illness are perceived by different classes, cultures and ages are perhaps more evident to GPs than to anyone else. A good GP should, by definition, recognise the delicate balance between mind, body and spirit in the treatment of his or her patients. It's not always easy to take all these multiple factors into consideration with our limited time and resources but most of us do try. We appreciate the importance of emotional factors in physical symptoms and that illness can affect patients, their families and their environments in a myriad of different ways. This patient who had turned her back on conventional medicine clearly felt let down by modern doctors. I personally won't be prescribing any alternative treatments, but I do think that I could learn a lot from the techniques and holistic approaches of many complementary practitioners.

Thai bride

As I mentioned in 'Who am I?' I love being an observer and sometimes playing a part in the soap operas that are people's lives. In real soap operas, the watcher can only shout at the telly when a character is clearly heading for a fall. As a GP, sometimes I have the opportunity to step in, but the problem is knowing whether it is the right thing to do. This was the problem I faced with John.

John had been my patient for a year or so. He was a nice enough bloke but struggled with poor social skills and he was also not particularly blessed in the good looks department. Perhaps unsurprisingly, he had reached his forties without ever having been in a serious relationship and so decided to go on a trip to Thailand to find a wife. I remember him coming to see me before his trip, nervously asking for advice on travel vaccines and malaria prophylaxis. Maybe I should have made the suggestion then that a two-week holiday to Bangkok was perhaps not the best way to find true love. However, I stayed quiet and a few months later John came to see me in order to register his new wife as a patient. Sung was 19. She was beautiful, elegant and also looked absolutely terrified. John looked like the cat who had got the cream. I can't imagine anything more frightening than being plucked from your family, friends and country, to be put into a cold, grey, unfriendly town with a much older and slightly odd man who was now your husband. She also barely spoke a word of English. Perhaps it was true love but I doubted it.

John was present during my first consultation with Sung. I asked Sung a question and when she looked at me blankly, John offered to help translate. I was impressed that John had learnt Thai, only to find that instead of translating my question into Sung's native language, he just repeated it in English but shouted in a slightly odd stereotype of a Chinese accent. It was like a Russ Abbot sketch from the 1980s.

After a few months, while her husband was at work, Sung started to learn English at a language school and took a part-time job in a burger bar with other students her age. It was not long after this that John came to see me with symptoms of painful discharge from his penis. I did a swab because I suspected chlamydia. Chlamydia can hang around undetected for a long time, but I didn't think that John had been anywhere near a woman for years until Sung came along. John had also proudly told me that Sung was a virgin when they got married. It seemed fairly obvious to me that Sung was sleeping around, but what did I tell John? When the results came back from his swab, I explained that chlamydia was a sexually transmitted infection and advised that Sung came in to be tested and treated as well. Despite them both having a course of antibiotics, John came back with another sexually transmitted infection not long afterwards. I tried to hint gently that these infections were probably coming from outside of the marriage but John simply couldn't accept that this could be possible. How much right did I have to interfere with this relationship? John was blinkered and in love. Sung was 19 and having fun with lads of her own age. I was watching this car crash unfold each week. If John were a friend, maybe I would have given him a shake and pointed out the obvious, but he wasn't a friend, he was my patient.

A few months later, Sung left John for a 20-year-old boy who played bass in a band. John was devastated and ended up on anti-depressants. 'Why didn't you tell me she was being unfaithful?' he blubbed. What could I say? My job was to point out the facts and hope that John reached his own conclusions. Perhaps I should have made those facts a little clearer.

Dead people

I've seen loads of dead people but I'm still quite scared of corpses. As a hospital doctor, one of my jobs was to go and certify death. During a night on call, I would be covering ten or more wards and be up most of the night doing odd jobs and reviewing sick patients. I recall one night when, after having just got to bed at about 4 a.m., my pager went off. The nurse on one of the geriatric wards told me that one of the patients had died. It was an expected death so although there was no resuscitation and CPR necessary, a doctor needed to certify the death before the body could be taken to the morgue.

It was a cold dark night and I had to force myself out of my warm bed to make the long trudge from the on-call room to the hospital. 'Room 12,' the nurse said as I wandered on to the ward. Rubbing the sleep from my eyes, I stumbled into the darkened side room. To certify death, a doctor has to ensure the patient isn't breathing, that his heart isn't beating, that his pupils are fixed and dilated and that he doesn't respond to pain. The pain response is usually elicited by rubbing your knuckles really hard on to the front of the person's chest. It is called a sternal rub. It hurts like hell and we also use it a lot on alive patients in A&E, as it wakes people from even the deepest drunken stupor. The room was dark and quiet and I was all alone with the body lying in the bed in front of me. Still half-asleep I decided to start with the pain response. As I pressed my knuckles hard on to the corpse's chest, it jumped up, grabbed my hand and let out an ear-piercing scream. This was soon joined by an equally loud and terrified scream that was being emitted by me. The nurse then flew into the room and said, 'Sorry, Doctor, did I say room 12? I meant room 10.'

Holistic earwax

Veronica Davis rarely came to see me as she favoured alternative medicine to the more conventional kind that I was attempting to practise. The very fact that she was in my consulting room that morning suggested that she must have been fairly desperate to have ventured in to see me.

'Hello, Ms Davis, how can I help you today?'

'I don't care what you say, I'm not seeing a surgeon. I won't let those barbarians invade me with their implements of torture.'

'I'm sorry, Ms Davis, but I'm not quite sure what the problem is.'

'I've got a serious ear problem, but I swear to God I'll die before you send me to one of those filthy disease-ridden hospitals. I know my rights. My body is my body and I'll be the one who decides if it gets chopped open, thank you very much.'

'First things first, let's have a look in that ear, shall we? Hmmm. Seems it is a bit blocked up with some earwax.'

'Does it need an operation?'

'No, I think some olive oil drops should do the trick.'

Ms Davis had clearly been expecting to have to fight me and 20 others off her as we forced her into a waiting operating theatre to be sliced open by some bloodthirsty surgeons. I don't have many friends who are surgeons and you won't often find me first in the queue to defend them, but I do think they are perhaps misrepresented sometimes. The alternative medicine brigade needs to realise that surgeons don't cut you open for fun. They would probably rather be playing rugby or getting very drunk and accusing each other of being gay. That is what they like doing best. They will only cut you open if they really have to. If you decide you don't want to be operated on, they will be only too happy to have one less patient on their ever-growing waiting lists. Very few surgeons are good at the touchy-feely sensitive stuff, but then us touchy-feely GPs would be rubbish at fixing a broken pelvis or repairing a burst aorta. You should see the mess I make trying to carve a roast chicken! We each have our skills and if it were me that was in need of an operation, I would happily put up with a slightly insensitive posh rugby boy if I knew that he was a good surgeon and could put me back together again.

Veronica had spent hundreds of pounds on alternative treatments for her ear problem before she came to see me. Neither the homoeopath, cranial osteopath, herbalist, nor Reiki practitioner had actually looked in her ear. If they had, they would have seen a whole lot of hard brown wax that looked pretty painful. It annoys me that alternative practitioners call themselves holistic without actually knowing how the body works. Surely that basic knowledge is as important a part of treating someone holistically as looking after their emotional and spiritual needs. I decided not to give in to the overwhelming desire to be smug with Veronica but instead just felt relieved that the consultation was drawing to a close with a simple diagnosis and simple treatment.

'But why has it happened?'

'Excuse me?'

'Why has the earwax formed? There must be a reason. Do you think it is because there has been an imbalance in my energies?'

'Erm, no. It just happens sometimes. I get too much earwax sometimes, too. Bloody annoying.'

'Well, perhaps, Dr Daniels, you're not facing up to some deep emotional issues that are being suppressed. Everything happens for a reason. You should look at your health more holistically.'

I'm all for trying to balance and integrate the physical, mental, emotional and spiritual aspects of disease, but this was earwax. *Bloody earwax!*

Obesity register

Jemma is 28 and has come to see me about an infected insect bite on her ankle. She is nice enough but not very confident and admits to feeling a bit nervous around doctors. We have a bit of a chat and I like to think that I put her at ease. Her bite needs some antibiotics and all is straightforward until my computer butts in. Flashing up on my screen is 'WEIGH PATIENT AND CONSIDER INCLUSION ON OBESITY REGISTER.' Yet another target in our target-based world. The computer wants me to weigh Jemma and if she is above a certain weight, I would be obliged to put her on a special register along with our other overweight patients. Hmm, how can I put this tactfully to Jemma?

'Oh Jemma, before you go, I've noticed you're a bit of a porker. Jump on the scales; mind not to break them now, cupcake. That's it . . . 16 stone. Bloody hell, you are a big girl! We're going to have to put you on our special fatties list. That's it, have a good cry. Maybe it will burn off a few calories. See you again soon for another weigh-in. Won't that be fun?'

Okay, so I am a little more subtle than that, but I do object to having to put my overweight patients on an obesity register. Perhaps I'm wrong here, but I imagine that a young woman would not want a young slim male doctor, whom she doesn't know, pointing out that she is overweight (something she is probably already aware of). Especially when she has come to see him about something completely unrelated.

Of course I recognise that obesity is a large problem with social and medical consequences. I sometimes have patients who come in to ask me specifically about their size and to seek advice and support about losing weight. When this happens, I'm happy to listen and try to offer some encouragement. I explain about eating less and exercising more, but generally the world is already over-saturated with information about losing weight. I don't really have that much more to add other than a sympathetic ear and a few supportive words.

Currently, we reach our target and get our points (and money, of course) by simply having patients on the register. We don't do anything with the register. There aren't teams of dieticians waiting to give advice and support to our overweight patients. There are no good slimming medicines that have been shown to significantly reduce weight in the long term. All in all, the list is currently fairly devoid of function other than successfully alienating a significant percentage of our patients. Perhaps we should make our obese patients wear a little yellow cake logo on their clothes so we can differentiate them from our 'normal' patients? Of course, I'm over-emphasising the point here, but I just feel that weight is a very sensitive subject and although encouraging healthy lifestyles is vital, are an enforced obesity register and regular weigh-ins the answer?

Dr Arbury

Dr Margaret Arbury is a GP and a formidable character. In my mind she is a cross between Mary Poppins and Margaret Thatcher. She is in her forties but has the air and dress sense of someone much older and from a different time altogether. Ultimately, she is very unlike the normal slightly fluffy, friendly female GP. As she opens her door to call in her patients, she ushers them in like an impatient schoolteacher. 'Come along, come along, Mrs Foster, one has other patients to see.' The patients are absolutely terrified of her and, as she puts it herself, she simply will not tolerate nonsense. Dr Arbury has never married and her real passion in life is horses. General practice seems an unlikely career choice for her and by her own admission she doesn't enjoy it, but it does enable her to spend a couple of days a week at work and the rest of the time at the stables.

There is a part of me that admires Dr Arbury's no-nonsense approach. She is a very good doctor clinically and is excellent at diagnosing and treating disease. She is not so good at doing the touchy-feely, sensitive stuff. Any sort of mental health issue tends to be treated with a 'pull yourself together'-type response and she prides herself at never giving out sick notes to the 'whining bone idle'.

There are some who respond well to her brutal but often reassuring honesty. 'Mr Evans, you are not dying of pneumonia, you have a cold, now stop making such a fuss and go home.' 'Thank you, Doctor. I was hoping you would say it was nothing serious.' If she decides that her patient is unwell, however, she will fight hand and tooth to get her/him the best treatment possible. I once heard some poor secretary trying to convince Dr Arbury that there would be a six-week wait until her patient could be seen by the hospital specialist. It didn't take long before Dr Arbury had the consultant on the phone and was instructing him on exactly when and where the appointment would take place. Getting to the point quickly means that she always runs to time, which is also popular.

The interesting thing for me is how many of the more difficult, needy patients respond well to her. One of my patients is an addict whose alcohol and Valium use I had been trying desperately to reduce for some time. To my amazement, she responded much better to being given a good telling off by Dr Arbury than by my softly-softly sensitive encouragement. The advantage of being a patient in a big practice is that you can choose the GP who suits you. As new GPs, we are often warned not to be too nice and fluffy or we'll get all the clingy needy patients latching on to us. Some difficult, needy patients often avoid seeing tough doctors like Dr Arbury because they don't get the sympathy and attention they crave. It sounds a bit patronising but sometimes I think that a firm word and some home truths can do us all a lot of good. Sometimes, my patients need a sympathetic ear and a bit of genuine empathy. At other times, like all of us, they need a good kick up the backside. The difficult part is getting the right balance.

Body fluids

Patients often take it upon themselves to bring in various samples of their body fluids for my perusal. I would like to emphasise that this is normally not appreciated. A pot of urine is generally not too bothersome. Often in a jam jar, I hold it to the light, stroke my chin and let out a 'hmmm'. I like doing this as it makes me feel like an old-fashioned doctor from the nineteenth century. Apparently, they were keen on diagnosing all sorts of illnesses by looking at the urine and then tasting it! Unlike a nineteenth-century doctor, I look but don't drink. I also hold back from prescribing leeches or a tonic of mercury, but instead dipstick the urine and usually offer some antibiotics for a urine infection. If you are going to use a jam jar to hold your urine sample, please wash it out first. I once tested a urine sample and broke the news to the patient that it was full of sugar and therefore a diagnosis of diabetes was possible. Fortunately for the patient, it turned out that the urine was full of sugar because the jar still had a bit of strawberry jam swimming around in it.

Other body fluids that have been brought to my surgery include:

1. A condom full of semen – the patient was worried that it was a funny colour.

2. Various samples of vaginal discharge on tampons and one miscarriage wrapped up in a tissue.

3. Lots of poo. One woman brought in a week's worth of her baby's soiled nappies. Each was neatly labelled with a time and date and she laid them out on my surgery floor in chronological order. 'As you can see, Dr Daniels, last Thursday morning is considerably more yellow and viscous in consistency than Saturday afternoon's.' I spend a lot of time convincing first-time mums it is normal for baby poo to be a bright mustard-yellow colour.

My only true body fluid aversion is sputum. I just can't bear the stuff. Every time I view sputum, I get a flashback to a particularly long ward round in which I was involved as a medical student. I was extremely hung over and after several hours of traipsing around hot and smelly wards, we finally got to our last patient, who I will call Mr Phlegming. He was an old guy with emphysema (knackered lungs from smoking) and spent his days coughing up gallons of sputum and collecting it to show us on the ward round. As we arrived, Mr Phlegming enthusiastically held out a plastic cup full to the brim with sputum. It had a plastic lid on it and clearly none of us including the consultant was particularly keen to examine its contents. Medics are a hierarchical lot and the pot got handed down from consultant to registrar, to senior house officer to house officer and then finally to me. As the medical student, I was clearly at the bottom of the food chain and as I held the cup in my hand it felt unfeasibly heavy. 'Come along, take a look,' my consultant barked impatiently. Opening the lid, I was greeted with a swirling mass of muck. Not quite green and not quite brown. Not quite liquid and not quite solid. It had a colour and physical state all of its own. I began to feel my stomach gurgle and then made my excuses, just reaching the toilet before spewing. Give me shit, piss, blood and vomit any day.

Racism

I'm meeting George for the first time. Everyone tells me how great he is. 'Good old George. He really is the salt of the earth. A retired docker. Always has a smile on his face. Brings us a tin of chocolates every Christmas. Everyone loves George.' After ten minutes with George I can't help but agree that he's a nice old boy. He's in his late seventies and, apart from a bad hip, he is basically fit and well. Cheery and friendly, we have a bit of a chat about the misfortunes of the local football team and he reminisces briefly about the good old days. After a bit of a look at his hip, I suggest that he might want to consider seeing the orthopaedic doctor as he could benefit from a hip replacement. 'Well, if you think it might help, Doc . . . One thing, though, I won't see no Paki doctor, will I?'

I hate it when this happens. You meet someone you think is nice enough and they turn out to be a raging bigot. It's so much easier to hate racists when they fulfil my expectation of being all-round arseholes. What do I do now? Do I confront a man in his late seventies about his life-long racist beliefs and try to re-educate him? Perhaps I could accidentally forget to make the referral? Some might argue that as patients are now encouraged to have 'choice' over which consultant they see, I should follow his request and find him the white British surgeon he wants. Remember it's not my job to judge, simply to treat and serve my patients to the best of my abilities.

'Some of my best friends are Asian doctors and they are also very good at their jobs,' I say firmly. 'If you want the referral to be made, then you'll get whichever doctor is allocated to you. We don't make allowances for racism.' George looks a bit taken aback.

'I'm not a racist or nothing. It's just I saw that Dr Singh bloke with my bad knee and I didn't understand a word he was saying.'

My friend Chirag is a GP and was born in Wembley to Indian parents. He has a London accent, is good-looking, dresses slickly and is a bit of a charmer. He is well liked by even some of his most hardened racist patients. My friend Anil, however, was born and brought up in India. He moved to the UK seven years ago after qualifying from medical school back home in Bangalore. Anil has a moustache, a side parting, unfashionable clothes and a thick Indian accent. He struggles to understand anyone with a strong regional accent and couldn't give a monkey's about beer, football or regional rivalry. He is a very good and dedicated doctor but the patients tend not to warm to him and he has suffered from quite a lot of active discrimination from both patients and staff.

The Georges of this world appear to have made some changes with regard to their racism. In my experience they are now more tolerant of the colour of someone's skin as long as the person speaks with a good British accent and can join in with a joke about Geordies or Scousers or the England football team. The other development is that patients tend to recognise that it is no longer acceptable to publicly verbalise their bigoted ideas, although they will still make a few sly racist comments if they think they can get away with them. I'll leave it to you to decide if these changes are any form of improvement or not.

It seems such a shame that racism has remained a deeply ingrained tradition of white working-class culture in certain parts of this country. Over the last 50 years or so overall prejudice has reduced and I think that the NHS has done more than any other institution to help transform racist ideas. There are a great number of different nationalities working within the NHS and has been for so many years that lots of people have had their only exposure to non-white people while going to hospital or seeing their GP. There is a story about an Indian GP who moved to a small Scottish Highlands town back in the 1960s. Initially, he and his family were met with some suspicion, but after a short period he became a much-loved member of the community and the attitudes of the local people were changed for ever.

Some people, unfortunately, are beyond help. I saw a fat middle-aged white man from the local estate who was requesting a prescription for some Viagra. He hadn't worked for years, citing his bad back, but his real disability was his enormous gut and the deep resistance he had to getting up off his sofa. I was happy to prescribe him some Viagra but explained that it wasn't available for free on the NHS and that he would be charged for his prescription. 'I bet the Pakis and immigrants don't have to pay, Doctor? You'd give me the pills for free if I was one of those asylum-seeking suicide bombers,' he retorted. I desperately wanted to point out that, first, it was unlikely that al-Qaeda make explosive suicide belts that would fit his enormous 64-inch waist and, second, that were anyone to demand a prescription while strapped with many kilograms of high explosives then, yes, I would undoubtedly write them the prescription of their choice completely free of charge. My reasoning for this would be my natural instinct to avoid getting myself blown up rather than because of a government policy that favoured non-whites as he appeared to be suggesting. I kept my mouth shut but did take great pleasure in writing out the private prescription, knowing that this racist heap of lard would have to pay for his erections while mine still came completely free of charge.

Sleep

Is not being able to sleep a medical problem? I'm not sure it is. I see lots of people telling me that they can't sleep and they want me to give them a cure. Usually, they ask for a sleeping pill and are then surprised by my reluctance to prescribe them one. We all have nights lying awake and watching the clock slowly tick by. It's not much fun but it strikes me as part of being human. Some people struggle more than others but usually we can find a reason for not sleeping. Causes can be divided into extrinsic and intrinsic. Extrinsic factors include having a crying baby or noisy neighbours keeping you awake. I can't do much about those, but intrinsic factors such as stress, anxiety, excitement and pain are probably more common causes of insomnia. There is usually something keeping us awake and I always feel that there are plenty of routes to explore before we make the knee-jerk reaction of reaching for the sleeping pills.

The problem with sleeping pills is that they are addictive and stop working after a short period. The manufacturers advise that they should not be taken for more than a month, but despite this I have literally hundreds of patients who have been taking sleeping pills for up to 40 years! Benzodiazepines (benzos) are still the most commonly prescribed sleeping tablet (aka Valium, diazepam, temazepam, etc.). For those patients on these medications, stopping them is extremely difficult. My patients on Valium are like any addicts. They crave their drug and will often lie, cheat and steal to make sure they don't miss their next dose. In the rougher parts of this country, Valium has a street value and is sold by drug-pushers along with heroin and crack cocaine. If it is viewed by dealers and junkies as an illicit drug, maybe it is time that doctors saw it in the same way.

Diazepam is a type of tranquilliser and works on specific receptors in the brain to relax muscles, relieve anxiety and cause sedation. In the short term it can seem like a wonder drug for all those angst-ridden insomniacs. The problem is the side effects. The body gradually gets accustomed to the sedative effect of the medicine and after a short period of time the drugs are no longer effective. Users start needing higher doses to have the same effect. They find that without the drug they feel increasingly anxious and unwell and can have quite severe physical side effects such as abdominal cramps, vomiting and even seizures. Taking sleeping pills at night often makes them feel slow and sluggish during the following day. I've had to sign people off work who were addicted to sleeping pills when they were too tired to work safely as a truck driver or machine operator during the day.

I'm not suggesting that we stop prescribing these medications altogether, as benzos do have their uses. They are valuable in calming and relaxing people prior to operations and if it wasn't for benzos, B. A. Baracas would never have got on a plane! They can also be used to bring epileptics out of a fit and I often prescribe them when someone is under acute stress. For example, in the immediate period after a bereavement or when a relationship has ended, a short course of diazepam can help someone to get through the first few terrible days. They are also good for patients with severe muscle spasm such as a slipped disc in the back.

I fully accept that there are drug and alcohol addicts out there. To add to those numbers many more addicts created by doctors, principally GPs, seems such a shame. There is still a strong culture of prescribing sleeping tablets among some GPs. It is the quick fix for both patient and doctor. The patient gets a pill that makes them feel relaxed and able to sleep and the doctor gets the patient out of the room quickly. It is much tougher for both patient and doctor to try to identify the underlying cause of the sleeping problem. Depression, pain and anxiety are all difficult issues and ten minutes isn't nearly enough time to handle them. For my patients who can't sleep, I usually ask why they think they can't sleep. I then move on to something called 'sleep hygiene' and offer advice about exercise during the day and having a hot bath and cocoa just before bedtime. I even add in a bit of feng shui and advise never to use the bedroom for anything other than as a place to sleep so that the bedroom tunes the brain into sleeping rather than thinking. Some patients like all this holistic stuff, others just want a magic pill and are disappointed when I say no.

Magic wand

My niece was five and for her birthday she got a pink fairy outfit that she insisted on wearing every day. The outfit came complete with a pink glittery magic wand, which, upon waving, lit up and made a '*didledidledidledidledeeee*' magic wand-type sound. I would love to borrow the fairy outfit and magic wand for some of my more difficult patients . . .

So, Kelly. Let me summarise, you're a 25-year-old single mum with three screaming children. You live in a cold, damp two-bedroom council flat and you've just had a big row with your mum and sister. It is a miserable wet day in late November and you've got no money for Christmas. You've been depressed for years and have already tried several different types of antidepressants but nothing has helped and today you've come to see me so that I can give you a pill to make you happy. Hold on, I'll just get my magic wand . . . *Didledidledidledidledeeee.*

So, Mr Jackson, you've been having headaches every day for 30 years. You've had multiple brain scans and blood tests and have been seen by three very good neurologists. A cause for your headaches has never been found and no medication has ever helped resolve them. You've come to see me today because you have a headache and want me to cure it . . . *Didledidledidledidledeeee.*

You have a cold and feel like shit . . . *Didledidledidledidledeeee.*

Of course, if I really had a magic wand, I wouldn't waste it on my heart-sink patients. There are much more important problems in the world to resolve:

Didledidledidledidledeeee . . . West Ham win the Premiership.

Didledidledidledidledeeee . . . Man United get relegated and Alex Ferguson cries on *Match of the Day*.

Didledidledidledidledeeee . . . Kylie lives next door to me but is otherwise unchanged.

Didledidledidledidledeeee . . . Kylie finally realises that she has always found slightly geeky, big-nosed doctors really quite attractive.

Didledidledidledidledeeee . . . Various other stuff involving myself and Kylie that I couldn't possibly put into print because my wife would kill me.

Okay . . . *Didledidledidledidledeeee* . . . World peace, end to poverty, reversal of climate change, etc. Yawn. Yawn.

Finally then I might find the energy to use my magic wand for the benefit of my heart-sink patients or I might just magic them off to another doctor.

I know that most of my patients with chronic health problems realise I don't have a magic wand or expect miracle cures. They want some of my time for support, reassurance and practical advice to help get them through difficult times. I'm quite happy to offer that but you'd be surprised about how many of my patients really do want a magic cure.

Didledidledidledidledeeee . . . My book outsells Harry Potter and I'm played by Brad Pitt in the Hollywood film adaptation.

Cannabis

Sometimes, even when my surgery is full, the receptionists sneak a couple of extra patients on to the end. Up on the screen next to their name is a little justification as to why they have been squeezed in. These might be: 'Baby with fever – mum worried' or 'Lost prescription – catching flight this afternoon.' After a recent busy afternoon surgery I had a 16-year-old boy added on to my list and the receptionist had put 'overdose' next to his name. I thought this was a bit odd, as normally the receptionists are fairly sensible and would send an overdose straight to A&E.

I called Adrian and his mum straight in from the waiting room. Adrian was dressed all in black and had long, straggly, greasy brown hair that covered his face. Despite trying to look gothic and alternative, Adrian still looked a lot more like Harry Potter than Pete Doherty. He did look pale and sickly but I was not sure whether that was the look he was trying to convey or whether he was actually unwell.

'He's taken an overdose, Doctor. Drugs! It's drugs!' Adrian's mum wailed with her head in her hands.

Mum was completely frantic and shouting and crying. Adrian was sitting awkwardly in the chair visibly squirming while staring at the floor. After a couple of minutes, I was getting nowhere as

Mum was hysterical and Adrian was monosyllabic so I politely asked Mum to wait outside. Once his mum had left the room, Adrian relaxed a bit and told me what had happened. He and his mates from his chemistry A level class had finished a mock exam and had gone to sit in the park to drink some cider. One of his mates had some cannabis and Adrian had tried some. Cider and cannabis don't mix very well so after three puffs, Adrian had started feeling a little pale and unwell, known in my day as 'pulling a whitey'. He had staggered home but, unfortunately, while on his way to his bedroom he had been intercepted by his mother. After a fierce interrogation, she had managed to force out of him that he had smoked some weed and then frantically dragged him straight to the surgery.

I brought Adrian's mum back in and tried to calm her down.

'Adrian's going to be fine,' I said.

'Well, doesn't he need some tests doing and his stomach pumped?'

'I promise that won't be necessary. He just needs to go home and get some sleep.'

'Well, what will happen now? Doesn't he need to go in for rehab? Won't there be some aftereffects?'

'Hmm, he might go and raid your fridge in about three hours but not much else.'

'Please tell him never to take drugs again, Doctor. He'll listen to you.'

Parents are very naïve if they think that their teenagers will listen to me. I am not one of those cool 30-year-olds who DJ at the weekend and wear product in their hair. I listen to Radio 4, grow tomatoes and lately have found myself remarking on how comfortable and practical a combination of socks and sandals is. Until recently, I thought the Arctic Monkeys were a result of climate change. Your children will quite rightly view me as a geek and will under no circumstances take any lifestyle advice from me. On numerous occasions I have been instructed by parents to lecture their teenage offspring on subjects varying from sitting up straight to eating more vegetables. It is embarrassing and pointless.

Adrian and his mum left and I felt embarrassed on his behalf. I'm not advocating drugs. They are bad and certainly cannabis is now known to be considerably more harmful than previously thought. Having said all that, teenage boys with long straggly hair will sit in the park and smoke weed. It has been going on since the 1960s and so long as there are parks and spotty teenagers, it will continue into the future. The vast majority of these boys will eventually realise that there are more interesting things to do in the world and wake up to the fact that long greasy hair and heavy metal T-shirts are a bad look. Their mates will then betray them in years to come by putting embarrassing photos of them looking stoned and dishevelled on Facebook.

Sick notes

These are some people who have asked me to sign them off work. What do you think? Would you sign them off?

A bloke in his late twenties works in some sort of IT firm. He has had a big row with his boss and has resigned, but doesn't want to work out his notice because the atmosphere is horrible in the office. He's a bit stressed about it all but isn't depressed or unwell and is out looking for new jobs and going to interviews. He wants a sick note to say he doesn't have to go to work for the next three weeks until his notice runs out. He won't get paid unless he gets one.

A woman has been on annual leave this week but has been in bed with a bad cold. She would like a sick note to say that she was unwell during her holiday so that she can take an extra week of annual leave at another time.

A 25-year-old bloke has been on jobseeker's allowance (the dole) for one year. Three months ago, he got really pissed, climbed a tree and then fell and fractured his leg, arm and pelvis. He is recovering quite well and is out of hospital but on crutches. If I give him a backdated sick note from when he had his accident, he can claim incapacity benefit for the time since his fall, which is more than jobseeker's allowance. Of note: he has spent most of the last three months being looked after in an NHS hospital and so has not really needed much money.

It is early November and a woman wants to be signed off on sick leave because Christmas is coming and her mother died at this time several years ago. Her cat has cancer and she thinks that she won't be able to cope at work until January. She doesn't have any symptoms of clinical depression.

A man was sacked from his job because of heavy daytime drinking and being drunk at work. He feels that he is unable to work now because of his alcohol dependence. He is not willing to be referred to an alcohol counsellor or a rehab programme.

A 25-year-old man was born with severely deformed arms and, at the age of 18, was signed off as disabled. A year ago he got a job at a supermarket but was sacked after being caught giving his friends unauthorised discounts. Now he wants to go back on to disability living allowance. He doesn't have any new illnesses or disabilities.

A 45-year-old woman who is extremely overweight and gets very short of breath because of her heavy smoking and large size. She did have a job in a supermarket but because it is on top of a hill she can't get there. She is making no effort to stop smoking or to lose weight.

What do you think of this lot? Would you sign them off? As you can see, the decisions I make on sick notes are often less related to my medical knowledge and more to do with my general sympathies towards a particular person on that particular day. When I hand out a sick note, I am basically signing that person a cheque made up of taxpayers' money.

Am I any more qualified to make these decisions than someone with no medical training? These patients are people doctors potentially know quite well and sometimes it can be hard to say no to them. It is also very difficult to prove or disprove what they are telling us. For example, I have a patient who tells me that she can't work because she has a panic attack every time she leaves her house. Perhaps she does. Perhaps she doesn't. I am not going to sit outside her house and follow her into town taking photos of her having a great time in a crowded shopping centre. Physical symptoms are equally difficult to disprove. If a patient tells me that he has back pain, who am I to disbelieve him? He may have multiple normal scans, X-rays and examinations, but if he tells me that his back hurts and he can't work, do I have the right to call him a liar? We are taught to listen to our patients and try to do our best for them. It is very difficult all of a sudden to start distrusting them and try to catch them out.

Although I do have patients trying to pull the wool over my eyes, most of my patients who are requesting a sick note or claiming disability payments are doing so genuinely. They have an illness or disability and need some medical documentation to verify this so that they can get some money to live on. Most people do actually want to return to work as soon as possible. Whatever our job, we generally moan about it and look forward to having some time off for a few weeks a year, but ultimately most of us want to be employed. It is partly how we define ourselves and there is a social stigma attached to not working. From a personal perspective, my job is rewarding and I feel valued. If I take time off, then I feel I am letting down my colleagues and patients. I do sometimes wonder whether my work ethic would be so strong if I had a less appealing job. If I toiled stacking shelves overnight in a supermarket for the minimum wage, I can imagine that the temptation for 'pulling a sickie' would be pretty strong. Perhaps I could even hoodwink my GP into writing me off work completely. I could then get close to the same pittance sitting at home on disability payments.

Most GPs hate giving out sick notes and filling in disability claim forms. They take up time and valuable appointment slots. I heard of one GP in a particularly deprived part of Wales who completely gave up trying to assess his patients' ability to work. He used to go into his crowded waiting room each morning and ask everyone who was in for a sick note to put up their hand. Without asking any of them a single question, he would then go round and dish out a sick note to each one of them and therefore clear half of his waiting room. This allowed him to spend his morning as a doctor rather than as a clerk for the Benefits Agency.

There are many millions of people on benefits and they are costing the country billions of pounds. As a GP, I have a social responsibility to try to encourage people to work. This is partly for the good of the national economy and also because working is good for you. Evidence shows that working is beneficial to our physical health and mental wellbeing. I wish I could convey this to some of my patients on long-term sick leave. Some of my 'disabled' depressed patients are only in their early twenties and I know that they'll probably never ever work. It is very sad and I don't want to sound unsympathetic, but moping around at home watching daytime TV surely can't be helping. When I have the energy, I do try to urge my patients to think about the positives of having a job and encourage them to get back to work. Sometimes, no matter how hard I try, they end up leaving with a sick note.

Drug reps . . . again

More of a moan about drug reps and the pharmaceutical industry's cosy relationship with some doctors. I need to point out that most GPs have a healthy mistrust of the drug companies. An average GP might see a pharmaceutical rep once a week or so to find out about the new drugs on the market, but they take the presented information with a pinch of salt and are able to make their own minds up about the best drug to prescribe for their patients and the country's health budget.

As I said earlier, most GPs now don't get much more of an incentive to prescribe a specific drug than the odd free pen or egg sandwich. However, one or two GPs are still very much in the tight grip of the pharmaceutical companies and exhibit what I feel are blatant unethical collaborations that are not in the best interests of the patient at all. The following events happened at a surgery where I once worked.

DEXA scanners are bone scanners that look for osteoporosis. This is a disease caused by thinning of the bones that can occur in people from middle age onwards and can contribute to the likelihood of breaking a bone, particularly in later life. The scanner measures how dense the bone is. For those people at risk of having thin bones, the scanner can identify those who might benefit from

219

taking calcium supplements and another type of medicine that can prevent bones from thinning further. These scans are available on the NHS and big studies have shown who is likely to be at risk and therefore which of our patients we should refer for scanning.

At the practice at which I was working, a drug company offered the senior partner a significant amount of money in order to allow them to scan our patients in the surgery with one of their mobile scanners. The mobile scanner is not as accurate as the big scanner that is available free of charge at the hospital. The senior partner phoned round many of her middle-aged, worried well patients and offered them a free scan at the surgery. Although they didn't fit the criteria for being at risk of having osteoporosis, most of them jumped at the chance to have a free scan that would be conveniently done at the surgery. They also had all heard of osteoporosis and wanted to ensure that they weren't at risk. The scanner appeared to overestimate how thin their bones were and therefore many of them were inaccurately diagnosed as having osteoporosis. These patients were then started on a medicine to keep their bones from supposedly deteriorating further. The senior partner was free to prescribe any medicine, but chose to prescribe the one that is made by the drug company that provided the scanner. This drug is considerably more expensive than other medications that are equally effective and costs the NHS £170 extra per year per patient.

I am very pleased to say that this sort of thing only still occurs in a very few practices and is being clamped down on. Our PCT has learnt a few tricks from the drug companies. We are still bribed to prescribe certain drugs but it is now the PCT that does the bribing. The practices in our local area are given targets to prescribe the cheaper drugs and if we hit the targets, we earn financial bonuses. This may seem crazy but the PCT have realised that for some GPs the only way to ensure that our drug spending is kept down is to reward us financially. The money they pay us for hitting the targets is nothing compared to the money saved by the NHS if we prescribe the cheaper generics. Yet again it feels embarrassing that doctors need financial incentives to prescribe sensibly.

Mistakes . . . I've made a few

I think medical errors can broadly be divided into four categories:

Type 1. The near miss: Making a mistake but it doesn't actually cause any harm to the patient.

Type 2. The cockup but arse covered: Missing a diagnosis and the patient comes to harm. However, the diagnosis was hard to make and the doctor did all the right things and documented this very well in the notes.

Type 3. The cockup and up shit creek: Same as the last category, but as well as missing a hard diagnosis and the patient coming to harm, the doctor didn't document things very well in the notes.

Type 4. The probably in the wrong job: Making a completely unforgivable mistake that can't really be excused regardless of the documentation. This might include refusing to examine a patient or repeatedly missing a really obvious diagnosis.

Thankfully, I have never made a mistake in type 4 and hopefully never will. To be fair, I actually think they are incredibly rare.

Unfortunately, I have made mistakes in the first three categories and although nobody really likes talking about their own mistakes, they are probably fairly typical of slip-ups made by young doctors like me so I thought you might find them interesting.

The near miss

As a very junior doctor I was on a ward round with my consultant and a final-year medical student. The consultant said that he wanted a transfusion for Mrs X and asked me to take some blood to send to the lab so that we could confirm which blood group she was.

After the ward round, I asked the medical student how confident he was in taking blood. He was happy to give it a go, so I asked him to go off and take some blood from Mrs X. He came back proudly ten minutes later with the blood and I labelled the forms and samples of blood and sent them to the lab. The next morning as we got to Mrs X on the ward round, she was sitting happily in her bed with her second bag of donated blood running through into her vein. My medical student suddenly turned very pale. 'Is that Mrs X?' he trembled. 'She's not the lady I took blood from yesterday. I took blood from that lady opposite.'

Now this could have been an absolute disaster. Giving the wrong blood group to a patient can make them very ill and potentially kill them. I had signed the form stating that the blood taken was from Mrs X and therefore would have to take responsibility for the error. The medical student should have checked who he was taking blood from but ultimately, I was responsible for supervising him so again the buck would have to stop with me. Fortunately, Mrs X and the patient from whom my dopey medical student did take blood had the same blood group so no harm was done. I plucked up the courage to tell my consultant what had happened. I was fully expecting the shit to hit the fan, but instead he stuck a fatherly arm round my shoulder and said, 'Don't worry, Ben, I made far worse mistakes when I was a junior. You got away with this one, but just make sure you learn from it and don't let it happen again.'

The cockup but arse covered

I saw a middle-aged man complaining of headaches. His headaches were fairly nondescript with no symptoms of weakness in his limbs or problems with his vision. He hadn't banged his head and the only thing of note was that he was feeling a bit tired and stressed out at work. I gave him a really thorough examination and documented everything very clearly in the notes, but basically reassured him that there wasn't likely to be a serious underlying cause of his headaches. A week later he was found collapsed at home and was found to have a brain tumour. His headaches were almost certainly related to this and I had missed it. However, during our consultation, I took him seriously and gave him a really thorough check-over. I also asked him to come back if his headaches weren't resolving. He is recovering slowly in a specialist neurology hospital after some quite major brain surgery.

The cockup and up shit creek

Some time ago I saw a woman with some odd tightness in her chest. She was well in herself and only in her mid-fifties. She told me that she had the symptoms when she went into town shopping and wondered whether they might be due to anxiety. I asked her lots of questions about the pain to make sure it didn't sound as if it was because of problems with her heart or lungs. I also gave her a thorough examination, but couldn't find anything wrong. I had a long chat with her about relaxation techniques and breathing exercises and told her to come back if the pain got worse. Three days later she collapsed with a heart attack. Again I had missed the diagnosis, but sometimes heart problems can present oddly and perhaps many other doctors would have done the same as me. In hindsight perhaps I should have done a heart scan and ordered some blood tests but these might not have made a huge difference. My real error in this case was that my documentation in the notes was really poor. I didn't write much about the pain she had or the examination I did. Legally, I hadn't covered myself at all.

As you can see, these three cases are all mistakes of sorts and could have landed me in trouble. As you can also see, the degree of the mistake doesn't always correlate with the amount of harm that comes to the patient. I have learnt a lot from them and I am a better doctor as a result. The near miss with the blood transfusion was probably the most negligent on my behalf yet as by pure good fortune no one came to any harm, I got away with it completely. Had things turned out differently, I could have been struck off and, much more importantly, the patient could have died.

Missing the brain tumour was the least negligent because I really did do a thorough well-documented history and examination. For the lay person reading this, you may feel that I should have sent the patient to have an urgent brain scan. Unfortunately, I don't have access to brain scans. My only option would have been to have sent him straight to A&E. As with most GPs, I probably see about 200 people per year complaining of a non-complicated headache. If all GPs sent all of these patients to A&E, the system would collapse. The wife of the headache man is considering suing me. I'm a little anxious about this, but I know that I am completely covered because I'm fairly sure that if 100 GPs read my notes, most of them would have done the same thing as me. I felt dreadful when I found out that I had missed that brain tumour, but without X-ray vision, I don't think I could have been a better doctor that day.

Confessions of a GP

Mistaking the chest pain for anxiety was similar to the headaches in that it was a difficult diagnosis to spot. However, if the patient had wanted to sue me she could well have been successful. I wrote so little in the notes from that consultation that if she had claimed in court that she had all the classic symptoms of a heart attack or angina, then I had nothing in writing to defend myself. Medico-legally if it isn't written down, it hasn't been done. Shortly after the heart attack, the patient came in with her husband to see me. They were angry and upset and wanted to know why I had missed the diagnosis. I made the excuse that it was sometimes difficult to spot heart-related chest pain, but ultimately I held my hands up and said sorry. The hospital cardiologist had fortunately told them that her presentation of heart pain had been very unusual and as he knew me from my days in the hospital, he backed me up by telling them that I was a very good doctor. As far as I know, my apology was enough and they are not planning any legal action.

If I miss a diagnosis, the patient suffers regardless. But from a legal viewpoint, irrespective of how excellent and thorough I was in the consultation, if I've not documented my findings, I may as well not have seen the patient at all. I see up to 40 patients per day so can't remember each consultation. Court cases often come up years after the incident occurs and the medical notes are often the only thing the doctor has to defend their actions. If something goes wrong, the patient will probably think that they have a vivid recollection of the consultation, but often the details of the event can change as the memory is recalled time and time again. An example of this is when a patient says, 'That Dr X told me I had a year to live' or 'The A&E doctor said I would never have children.' First, doctors rarely commit to these sorts of bold statements and second, when I read the notes from those consultations, the documentation tends to be very different from the patient's recollection.

227

It is quite hard for a doctor to admit mistakes and I think what I'm trying to say here is that although I'm not the best doctor in the world, I'm mostly quite a good doctor. Mistakes happen to all of us. I try my best each day to avoid missing any serious health problems but I have made mistakes in the past and undoubtedly will make them in the future. My only other option would be to refer every headache I see for an urgent CT scan and every chest pain to A&E for a hospital admission. Perhaps in an ideal world I would do this but the NHS wouldn't cope with the strain and it would also cause unnecessary anxiety to many well people.

Some mistakes are genuinely because of negligence by poor doctors. Most mistakes are made by good doctors who perhaps missed a difficult diagnosis or didn't write enough in the patient's notes. I hope we don't become like the USA where ambulances are chased by lawyers hoping to persuade unwell people that it could be their doctor who is to blame for their illness. On the other hand, were it my family member who was ill or dead because of a possible medical error, perhaps I would want some justice too.

Dying

Our frequent close proximity to death and dying is perhaps one of the features that sets doctors apart from people in other professions. For most people, death is fairly sanitised now. It is rarely seen in its gritty reality and many people of my generation will never have seen a corpse or even somebody very ill. The constant exposure to something that most people would find very shocking can't help but take its toll on your personality and outlook on life. Of course, we don't suddenly acquire these characteristics upon passing our final medical school exams. Death and dying become gradually normalised as we are processed through the system of medical school and our first hospital jobs as junior doctors. In our very first week at medical school, we were cutting up corpses in the dissecting room. This was partly to learn anatomy, but also an attempt to give us an early exposure to death and help us learn to distance ourselves from it emotionally. I know that I must have normalised dying in my head because, although I have seen hundreds of people die, I can only actually remember one or two of them. Perhaps I'm particularly callous or have an exceptionally bad memory, but as I'm sitting here now racking my brains, I can recall very few of the names or faces of patients whom I have watched breathe their last breath.

Although I now feel very unsentimental towards death, the first patient that I watched die is etched very strongly in my memory. I can picture her face very clearly and I can even remember her name but I'll call her Mrs W. She was an ordinary 60-year-old woman who had woken up as normal that morning. She had felt fine and had been getting herself ready for what she had expected to be a fairly average day. Somewhere between breakfast and getting ready to pop to the post office, her aorta burst. The aorta is the main artery that runs from the heart, so as you can imagine having it spring a leak is bad news. It was my first hospital attachment as a medical student and I was hanging around A&E trying to learn something and not get in the way. As a third-year medical student, I was in a strange void between being a normal person and being a doctor. I'm fairly sure that no other nurse or doctor who was working that day will have any memory of Mrs W because it would have been just another day at work. But for me, it was all very new and shocking and I still remember the episode in distinct detail. I was seeing death in the way a non-medical person might see it and not from the perspective of the hardened doctor that I am now.

When Mrs W's aorta ruptured, she had a sudden pain in her abdomen spreading to her back and began to feel faint. She called an ambulance and after the casualty doctor felt her tummy and saw her blood pressure dropping, it became fairly clear that she had burst her aorta (known as a ruptured AAA – abdominal aortic aneurism). She needed an emergency operation and there were all sorts of people flapping around organising scans and getting the operating theatre ready. As a medical student, I had the advantage of not having my own role or job to do. I could just sit with the patient and take it all in.

During the following ten minutes, several more doctors arrived, prodded her tummy and spoke among themselves. Despite being very unwell, Mrs W had been alert and conscious through the whole ordeal. Nobody had really had the chance to tell her what was going on, but from the commotion occurring around her it was obvious that things were serious. She lay in bed connected to drips and monitors, yet stayed calm and immensely dignified. Her husband and daughter were sitting on either side of the bed, each holding one of her hands. The consultant surgeon soon arrived on the scene. He was a big burly man and was already in his surgical blues as he barked instructions at the nurses and junior doctors. I felt a pang of fear just by being in his presence. He marched over to Mrs W, sat down at the side of the bed and took her hand.

'I'm Mr Johnson and I'm going to be operating on you this morning. You have burst the main blood vessel that runs from your heart. If we don't fix it, you'll die. If we do an operation, there is a 50 per cent chance that you will survive.'

The words on paper look unbelievably harsh but Mr Johnson spoke them with an amazing air of calm and gentleness. He refused to be distracted by the surrounding mayhem but instead focused all his attention on Mrs W and her family. Sitting and watching, I was overcome with an amazing sense of how her life lay so tightly in the balance. She could sit up and talk and see and hear, but hidden beneath her skin, she was slowly bleeding into her abdominal cavity and ultimately dying.

'It is a major operation and we will need to replace the part of the burst vessel with a synthetic tube. After the operation, you may be in intensive care for some time. We're going to wheel you into surgery and start operating straight away. Do you have any questions?'

Mrs W and her family shook their heads. As the porter came to wheel her into surgery, she took back the hands of her daughter and husband. I assumed that she would say goodbye, tell them how much she loved them or at least leave them with some poignant words. Instead, she listed a series of instructions. 'There's some mushroom soup in the fridge that needs using up and your dad is running low on his athlete's foot powder. I owe the window cleaner from last week and don't forget to send a card to your auntie June on Tuesday, as it's her birthday . . .' The list of non-essential instructions continued right up until the anaesthetist put her to sleep. I wanted to shake her and say, 'Don't you realise what's happening? This might be the last time you see your husband and daughter! Don't you want to say goodbye?' I guess we all deal with things differently and this was the way that Mrs W dealt with what must have been an overwhelming and bewildering experience.

I changed into surgical blues and went into theatre. About halfway through the operation, Mrs W's heart stopped. It was bizarre watching them do CPR on her chest when her abdomen was lying wide open. Her heart never restarted. The surgeons changed out of their surgical clothes, told her family the bad news and then carried on with their day. I imagine they barely gave her death another thought.

I, on the other hand, was quite upset by Mrs W dying. It played on my mind for several weeks and I thought about her a lot. She was the first patient that I had watched die and although she was ultimately a stranger, I felt quite upset. I have never felt that way since about a patient dying. Sometimes I wish I could get that fresh and almost innocent compassion and emotion back. In some ways it would probably make me a more empathic and caring doctor, but at the same time if I felt like that about every patient who died, I would have had to give up the job years ago.

Happy pills

In one surgery I worked in, 1 in 10 of the adult patients was on antidepressants. That seems a huge number to me! I'm not sure if we were overprescribing them, or if our patients were a particularly miserable lot. I am certainly no expert in this subject, but depression is something that I see a huge amount of in general practice. The vast majority of cases are dealt with by us rather than psychiatrists and most GPs have had to become skilled in recognising the symptoms of depression and offering support.

Depression used to be a subjective diagnosis based on the outlook of the doctor and the patient. The powers that be seem to find this a difficult concept so have found ways for us to measure depression. This allows us to fit the depressed patient into a neat box and follow a set protocol. The result is that we can then be measured and shown to be either achieving or failing to reach targets. I find this very irritating. Many people with depression don't ever seek help. It takes a lot for a person to find the courage to come and see a doctor and tell him or her about some very difficult thoughts and feelings that they may be experiencing. It is a very personal consultation and usually requires the doctor to mostly listen and occasionally ask a few questions that may help elicit a few of the more subtle issues and personal aspects of the illness.

I like to think that after having worked in psychiatry and now having been a GP for some time, I'm quite skilled in this area. Unfortunately, in order to reach targets and hence earn points and money, I now have to interrupt a potentially very sensitive and important consultation to fill in a questionnaire. The answers give me a number by which the computer can categorise the person's feelings and decide whether they need an antidepressant or not. I find this slightly demeaning to both me and the patient.

My other big issue with the way GPs treat depression is the automatic reflex we seem to have for giving out antidepressants. I am certainly not against antidepressants and feel that for many people they play a valuable role in helping improve lives, but are we overprescribing them? For me, there seem to be three common presentations of depression that we see day in and day out in general practice. The symptoms can be quite similar, but I feel that the underlying cause can be very different and that this is fundamental to how we treat it.

Type 1. Grieving

You don't have to be a doctor to know that if something bad happens to us we feel sad. A bereavement or a relationship breakdown can give us all symptoms of depression. Feeling tearful, poor appetite and problems sleeping are all classic examples. Using my questionnaire, these symptoms would flag up a diagnosis of depression and suggest antidepressants, but is this really the right diagnosis? Isn't a grief reaction a normal part of being a human? I'm not saying that these patients shouldn't come to see their GP. We can offer support and a sympathetic ear. Maybe we could even refer them for counselling, but in the majority of cases, time and support from family and friends are enough to get people through these difficult times. Isn't it okay to feel sad sometimes?

Type 2. Classic clinical depression

These people often spend much of their lives moving in and out of long bouts of depression. The condition severely disables the sufferer and those close to them and is a diagnosable 'illness'. Often there is a strong family history of the disease and although there may be triggers for depressive bouts, sometimes there is no obvious cause and from the outside the sufferer has absolutely nothing to be depressed about. There is a risk of suicide and these people often do benefit from medication. The antidepressants alter the way in which certain neurotransmitters work in the brain and, sometimes along with other types of support, can help people turn the corner and begin to feel better.

Type 3. Low-grade misery

This is probably what I see most of when working in an inner city. I spoke earlier in this book about TLS – tough life syndrome. This is the theory that people are suffering from symptoms of depression but rather than an imbalance in certain brain chemicals, they are simply living a really hard and often shitty life. This may seem like a harsh derogatory generalisation, but I defy anyone who works with single mums on the council estates of this country to deny that TLS exists. Yet again, my computer's questionnaire labels these patients as depressed, but I generally find antidepressants fairly ineffective in these cases. For example, I saw a young single mum who had been feeling miserable for years. She wanted to try yet another happy pill and was demanding to know why none of the previous antidepressants had worked. Rather than just sign another prescription, I decided to try a new approach. We went through all the reasons that she felt miserable. These included being abused as a child, never knowing her father and having a difficult relationship with her mother. She had had abusive relationships with several men as an adult and and as a result was now alone with three children. She was unhappy with her appearance, had no confidence in herself and was struggling financially. She lived in a small, damp council flat in a particularly rough estate with lots of crime. Reflecting on all the shit things in her life didn't exactly lift her mood but then we made a list of positive things for her to attempt. She is now doing a college course and claiming for child support from her children's fathers. A small step, but more mood lifting than a little white pill.

People feel low for all sorts of reasons and whatever they are they should still come and see their GP for support. The point I'm trying to make is that one size doesn't fit all. Maybe we should try harder to look for alternative ways of helping people rather than always simply trying to make all the bad stuff disappear with a happy pill. Some people benefit from counselling or other forms of talking therapy, although, unfortunately, these are generally very oversubscribed and underresourced. Some people don't actually want counselling or antidepressants but simply feel a bit better by coming to see me and telling me that they are feeling a bit sad. It can feel odd as a doctor not to then prescribe something or make a referral. It feels like I'm not doing anything at all but I've learnt not to underestimate the healing power of simply listening.

Top 1 per cent of the population

These are apparently genuine excerpts from medical school entrance exams.

1. Three kinds of blood vessels are arteries, vanes and caterpillers.
2. Blood flows down one leg and up the other.
3. The hookworm larvae enters the human body through the soul.
4. For fainting: rub the person's chest or, if a lady, rub her arm above the hand instead.
5. For fractures: to see if the limb is broken, wiggle it back and forth.
6. For dog bite: put the dog away for several days. If he has not recovered, then kill it.
7. For nosebleed: put the nose much lower than the body.
8. For drowning: climb on top of the person and move up and down to make artificial perspiration.
9. To remove dust from the eye, pull the eye down over the nose.
10. For head colds: use an agoniser to spray the nose until it drops in your throat.

11. For snakebites: bleed the wound and rape the victim in a blanket for shock.
12. For asphyxiation: apply artificial respiration until the patient is dead.
13. Before giving a blood transfusion, find out if the blood is affirmative or negative.
14. If the lady is sexually activated, you must do a pregnancy test.

Computers

I was on holiday in Namibia. I was sitting around a fire in one of the most remote deserts on earth, yet simply by using my mobile phone, I could instantly view photos of my cousin's new boyfriend in Australia and read a full and detailed report on how my Sunday league football team had lost again in my absence. Once back home in NHS land if my patient goes to see a consultant at the hospital two miles down the road, I have to wait several weeks for his letter to be typed, posted, arrive at my surgery and then be filed by my secretary. It seems crazy to me that we are so backward when it comes to something as essential as sharing important information about patients.

In general practice our failure to have embraced technology is usually nothing more than an annoyance, but in hospitals it can be more than that. Currently, if an unconscious patient is admitted to A&E in the middle of the night, the doctors will often have very limited medical information about them. The patient might have some paper notes in a file sitting in a secretary's office somewhere, but unfortunately, there is no way that the A&E doctor can access the GP's computer records, which might have lots of very useful information that could potentially help save the patient's life.

If A&E had access to the medical records, we might have information that s/he was a diabetic or a heroin addict or even that s/he had advanced cancer and didn't want to be resuscitated. As you can imagine at 3 a.m. on a Sunday, this information could be very useful and greatly increase the speed with which we could make a diagnosis. The records might also give us a relative's telephone number and a list of the person's normal medication.

There are obviously big benefits of having all our medical records on a computer system to which all healthcare professionals can have access. The area that many people are concerned about is maintaining confidentiality. There are so many people working for the NHS and in social care that sensitive personal information about us all could be available to a huge number of people. For example, if my sister up in Newcastle started seeing a new bloke, might it be tempting for me to look up his healthcare records? Unethical as it would be, I could find out if he had ever had genital warts or been arrested for hitting his ex-wife. These are the sorts of personal details that are often on our medical records and access is currently only available to the staff at your current practice.

Presently, the government is investing billions into a new integrated computer system for the NHS. The plan is that we will be able to store patients' records centrally and also send referral letters and book appointments online. We are nowhere near having the system fully in place yet, but there have already been the usual grumbles of discontent. This has partly been because of criticisms about the quality of the technology and also opposition from patients and doctors. Personally, I do think that we do need to update the way in which we work. The technology would be a huge time-saver and, in some cases, a life-saver. Somehow we need to maintain patients' trust and perhaps do this by allowing them to keep certain parts of their records excluded from the national database. The worst possible outcome of a national computer system would be that patients no longer felt safe disclosing personal information to their doctors.

Kieran

Perhaps the most influential thing that happened to me at medical school was the death of a close friend. Kieran and I did our A levels together and as I went off to medical school, he had gone off to Leeds to start a psychology degree. Towards the end of my first year, I got a phone call from Kieran saying that he was in the hospital attached to my medical school. He had discovered a lump in his armpit some time ago, but full of the excitement of his first year at university, it had taken him a while to get round to seeing his GP. He was quickly diagnosed with a type of cancer called non-Hodgkin's lymphoma.

Over the next two and a half years, Kieran proceeded to have several courses of radiotherapy and chemotherapy for his cancer. He had periods of remission but, unfortunately, they were always followed by a relapse. Our worlds had always been very similar, but now they seemed far apart. I would sit in lectures learning about the side effects of chemotherapy and just a few floors above me Kieran was lying in a hospital bed losing his hair and vomiting his guts up. I used to pop in to see him between lectures and even wheeled him, drip in tow, into our student union bar to watch a few of the big England games during the 1998 World Cup.

Kieran came from a big Irish family. During my teenage years, I had spent a lot of time at his house and I knew his parents well. There was no one medical in his family and during Kieran's treatment his parents clung to me as a source of medical knowledge and as someone to translate the jargon into real English. I didn't really want this role. I was only a couple of years into medical school and hadn't even heard of non-Hodgkin's lymphoma when Kieran told me he had it. I wanted to be there simply as Kieran's friend and wasn't ready to play the role of doctor during this awful illness.

As I progressed through medical school, Kieran's cancer spread and worsened. I learnt more medicine and did begin to gain a limited understanding about some of the medical components of his illness and treatment. Eventually, the cancer spread to his brain and although Kieran and the rest of the family seemed to view this as only a minor setback, my basic medical knowledge was sufficient to know that the prognosis was now very poor. Just after Christmas 1999, Kieran declared that he had been given the all clear. He hired out a bar and threw a big party to celebrate. Kieran still looked terrible but told everyone it was simply the aftereffects of his chemotherapy. Deep down I knew that something wasn't right but I so wanted him to be cured that I let myself believe that he was. While his friends got drunk and partied, Kieran sneaked off home and took a massive overdose. He had been told earlier that week that his cancer was now untreatable but he clearly didn't feel able to tell us this. He wanted to have a big party and then go out with a bang. I guess he needed to take back some control over his life that had been ruled by the cancer for so long.

Kieran's overdose was unsuccessful and he had two more precious weeks before he died peacefully at home. He had the opportunity to say goodbye to family and friends, plan his funeral and decide where he wanted his ashes to be scattered. We were all grateful for those last weeks and I hope Kieran was, too. At his funeral I remember his mum hugging me and, as we both wept she said to me, 'This will make you a better doctor.' An amazing thing to be said by a woman who had just lost her 22-year-old son. I just hope she was right.

Peter

''Allo, Doc. We've got a right one for you 'ere. Mad as a box of frogs. We found 'im running down the middle of the dual carriageway completely starkers and shouting in gobbledygook.'

It was 3 a.m. on a cold February night and I was on call for psychiatry. The police had picked up my latest patient and, after diagnosing him with being 'as mad as a box of frogs', a common police diagnosis, they kindly dropped him off at the psychiatric ward for me to assess. The man, who we later found out was called Peter, was in his early twenties and looked fairly frightened. He was shouting in an unfamiliar language and was miming being attacked and chased. He gave the policemen each a hug (very much unappreciated) and they left him in my less than capable hands. Peter was wrapped in a blanket kindly donated by the local constabulary and given how cold it was outside, I wondered quite how he had survived any length of time being completely nude out on the dual carriageway in the middle of nowhere.

The most likely diagnoses going through my mind were some form of paranoid psychosis, possibly drug induced or maybe schizophrenia. He may have been having some form of manic episode but without him seeming to understand a word of English, the assessment was very difficult. We sat in a quiet room and I tried in vain to communicate, as did he, but we got nowhere. He had no clothes, no wallet and absolutely nothing to identify himself with. I admitted him to the psychiatric ward. What else could I do?

The next morning, I took my consultant to see him. Peter was a bit calmer, but still gesticulating and shouting. My consultant tried speaking to him in French, which gave me the giggles as it just made an odd consultation even more ridiculous, especially as my consultant's French was terrible and the patient was clearly from Eastern Europe somewhere. We do have interpreters available but we had no idea where this guy was from so didn't know where to start. After nearly an hour of getting nowhere, Ludmila, the ward's Polish cleaner, came into the room to empty the bin. The patient took one look at Ludmila and then said a few words to her and gave her a smile and a wink. Despite the language barrier, it was obvious to us that Peter was speaking the international language of leering and bad pick-up lines. Ludmila gave him an icy look and turned to us. 'He is of Belarus. He is not mad, just drinking too much wodka. Always the same is man from Belarus. Too much drinking, gambling and chasing of womans. Not enough working. They have bad reputation in my country.'

My consultant looked annoyed. 'Ludmila, do you actually speak his language?'

'No, just recognise he is of Belarus. All men from there are the same. Not mad, just drunk.'

'Thank you, Ludmila, but perhaps it might be best to leave the psychiatric diagnosis to me.'

Ludmila shrugged, gave Peter another icy stare that made the whole room shiver and left. We phoned up the interpreting service and found out that it was going to be five days before a Belarusian translator would be available. We still weren't sure if he was having paranoid delusions and needed some form of psychiatric medication. He had no money and didn't seem to know anyone here so we kept him on the acute psychiatric ward. Most of our young male psychiatric patients spent their time on the ward sleeping, eating, watching TV and occasionally masturbating. Peter was like a breath of fresh air. He enthusiastically joined in the ward's activities, going to the cooking morning, creative-painting day and Sunday morning yoga class. He also didn't let his failure to be understood prevent him from trying all his favourite Belarusian chat-up lines on the female patients, staff and visitors.

Eventually, the translator arrived and we crowded into the interview room to finally conduct a proper consultation. Peter launched into a long monologue in Belarusian and, with the help of the interpreter, we were finally able to find out a bit more about how Peter had ended up on our ward.

It turned out that Peter had arrived in England the previous week to find work and make some money. He met some Lithuanians at the coach station and they said that they could find him some work on a farm picking cabbages. To celebrate his first night, they played cards and drank vodka. He got very drunk and remembers losing his money and then his clothes in the game. He didn't remember much else but thinks he then got into a fight with one of the Lithuanians and they chased him naked from the farm. He was a bit cold but he assured us it was nothing compared to Belarusian winters. The police picked him up after an hour or so and he was very impressed that they were kind and didn't beat him. He also thanked us explicitly for our kind hospitality during his stay. He found that English people were very nice but some of the residents here were a little strange. He had decided to return to Belarus, as travelling wasn't really his thing. He then invited us all to stay at his home at any time and told us that we would all be made very welcome. Apparently, his mother made the best goulash in the whole village. Peter gave us each a kiss on both cheeks and left. I dread to think how much it cost the NHS to keep him on an acute psychiatric ward for five days but probably more than Peter could earn in a year back home. Ludmila was very smug. 'Like I am saying, all Belarus man the same. Lithuanians man even worse.'

Granny dumping

Granny dumping is the act of getting your elderly relative admitted to hospital in the build-up to Christmas so that the rest of the family can have a less stressful holiday period. I remember the more senior doctors moaning about granny dumping in the build-up to my first Christmas after I qualified. I didn't believe that it could actually happen, but every year before Christmas there is an influx of elderly patients whose families can't cope with them any more or who are jetting off to a converted farmhouse in Tuscany that doesn't have a stairlift.

Granny dumping is a very harsh expression and the actual individual cases are more complex. Being a full-time carer for a family member is an immensely difficult and often thankless task, but crises always seem to occur at Christmas and all too often lead to an unnecessary hospital admission. This is exactly what happened to one of my elderly patients one Christmas Eve. I was covering the afternoon session at a small surgery where I didn't know the patients. It was nearly 6 p.m. and I was looking forward to getting home to start celebrating Christmas with my family.

The phone rang as I was just seeing my last patient of the day. A distraught daughter was crying down the phone: 'It's my father. We can't cope any more. He's got Alzheimer's and he's getting

251

frailer. My mother had a stroke two years ago and can barely look after herself. We need some help.'

'It's 6 p.m. on Christmas Eve,' I unhelpfully pointed out.

'I know!' wailed the daughter. 'I've got my own family to look after and my sister is away skiing. Dad gets confused during the night and wanders around the house. He just needs someone to sit with him overnight. Someone to make sure he doesn't fall. My mother can't be expected to do it, she's too frail. I've got my daughter and her young family staying at ours so I can't do it myself. If you can't arrange something, he'll have to go into hospital.'

I hate these situations. I was being made to feel responsible for this person's difficult situation. It wasn't fair to admit him to hospital when he wasn't actually unwell; however, I could see the daughter's viewpoint. She had her own family to look after and didn't want to spend Christmas Eve chasing her confused father around his house. What I couldn't understand is why this always seems to happen just before the holidays start. Couldn't something have been organised weeks ago?

This was a social problem rather than a medical one. Other than take him back to my house and have him spend Christmas with me, I didn't really know what I could do. I 'Googled' the telephone number for the local emergency social services and gave it to the daughter. I told her that they might be able to organise some sort of emergency care overnight. Her dad didn't need a qualified nurse, just a caring person to sit with him and guide him back to bed when he got up and started wandering. There were enough carers in this town who would probably appreciate the money and plenty who weren't Christian and would happily work on Christmas Eve.

Half an hour later I phoned the daughter back to see how she had got on. She told me that she had dialled the number I had given her but no one had answered. After ten minutes she called 999. The ambulance had just taken her dad to A&E.

Another Christmas granny dump delivered to the NHS. Once in A&E on Christmas Eve, there was no way that he would get home. The cost of the ambulance, A&E treatment and ward admission would be thousands of pounds and I just hoped he didn't get a bout of MRSA with his hospital mince pies. Someone sitting with him overnight would have not cost more than £100. What a waste.

Some areas have wonderful emergency social services with a team of physios, carers and social workers on call to provide urgent assessments and vital care to people who desperately need it. They keep people out of hospital, saving money and preventing people from catching MRSA and other hospital bugs. Unfortunately, most emergency social services teams are terribly underfunded, under-staffed and suffer from low morale. They might not have a flashing blue light on their cars but they are desperately needed and would pay for themselves many times over by preventing unnecessary hospital admissions, especially at Christmas.

Ed

Medics' humour can be fairly brutal and one of our favourite games was stitching up our mates. Ed was a friend from medical school but when the rest of us qualified, he failed his exams and the poor bugger had to retake. Six months later, he did qualify and came and joined us as a hospital doctor. Ed was taking over my job on the ward and was extremely nervous about his first day. As I left on my last evening, I had the ward in fairly good shape ready for Ed to take over in the morning. However, we thought it might be entertaining to fish out a few embarrassing photos of Ed from medical school. Using the ward computer, we put a particularly unflattering photo of Ed on a notice. It stated: 'THIS MAN CLAIMS TO BE A DOCTOR CALLED DR EDWARD BENNETT. HE IS A CONMAN. PLEASE REPORT HIM TO SECURITY IF SEEN ON THE PREMISES.' We put the notices up on the ward that he was due to start on the next morning and then left for our new placements at different hospitals. Poor old Ed spent his entire first morning having to try to prove that he was really a doctor and eventually had to ask the dean of the medical school to confirm his identity.

Poor Ed was eventually allowed to start work and he survived his first year as a doctor. His next job was as a casualty doctor and, unfortunately, his first day was equally disastrous. We have a system where, at the beginning of August, we all swap jobs overnight. Often a doctor will be on call in one hospital one evening and then start work in a hospital in a different part of the country the next day. This is what happened to Ed. After finishing a shift at midnight, he woke up at 4 a.m. to drive 100 miles to a new hospital to start work in A&E. Ed didn't know the area and was driving around town lost, trying to find the hospital. Unfortunately, the combination of being sleep-deprived and lost resulted in him crashing his car on a roundabout. He wasn't badly hurt but the paramedics wanted to play things safe and he was wheeled into the A&E department where he had been due to start work, strapped to a spinal board and wearing a neck brace.

Being ill as a doctor is always a difficult experience, especially if you end up being admitted to the hospital in which you work. During my first year as a doctor, I was admitted for an operation on my ankle. It was very odd being on the other side and quite an eye-opener. My friends, of course, saw it as an excellent opportunity to stitch me up. They managed to find my drug card and thought that it would be hilarious to write me up for all sorts of unnecessary medications that would mostly have to be inserted up my backside. Still dopey from the anaesthetic, I had to fend off a particularly enthusiastic Filipino nurse who was determined to carry out all the doctors' carefully written instructions.

Camouflage man

Camouflage man is frightening when you first meet him. He has a big bushy beard and wears head-to-toe army camouflage gear, complete with balaclava and army cap. He is homeless and carries all his belongings in a large holdall on his back that he secures to his body with a long chain that is wrapped around him several times and locked with a big padlock. Camouflage man has paranoid delusions that he is being followed and people are trying to attack him and steal from him. These thoughts are partly because of his mental illness and partly because life on the street is tough and he regularly gets beaten up and robbed. You would probably cross the road if you saw camouflage man walking towards you, but now that I know him I realise that he is much more afraid of you than you are of him. His real name is Nigel.

Nigel is mentally ill but because he doesn't fit nicely into one neat category of mental illness, no one has really taken responsibility for him. Nigel has had schizophrenia since he was a teenager but because he is also an alcoholic and homeless, no one is very sure which team should be looking after him. Nigel won't take any medication and won't attend any psychiatric appointments. He often disappears for a few months at a time, but he always resurfaces and as his GP, I am perhaps the only healthcare professional with whom he regularly has contact.

He often tells me about his psychotic and frightening thoughts. They have been going on for years and are worse when he smokes cannabis. He sometimes becomes violent when he drinks and he has spent some time in prison. You might think that someone like Nigel should be in a psychiatric hospital and, 20 years ago, that is where he would have been. However, people with mental illness aren't locked away indefinitely these days as they are treated in the community instead. Care in the community works well for some people with mental illness, but not for Nigel. He is a 'revolving-door' patient. He becomes quite mentally unwell and often then ends up being compulsorily detained by the police and brought into hospital. He is forcibly given a drug- and alcohol-detox along with antipsychotic medication. For a period of time, he remains relatively well, but he can't be locked up for ever and eventually he is discharged and goes back to his old addictions and stops taking his medication.

My main worry with Nigel is that one day he might get very paranoid and kill somebody. It is very rare for somebody with mental illness to commit murder, but it does sometimes happen and when it does, the debate on how we should manage people like Nigel is reopened. The finger is pointed at GPs, psychiatrists and politicians and then everything blows over and not much changes. Today we can't lock up Nigel because he isn't harming himself or anyone else. I am scared that if he smokes enough dope, he might get sufficiently paranoid to harm someone, but my fears aren't a good enough reason to lock him away. Nigel does have a designated psychiatric nurse, who is very nice but struggles to keep track of him. There are only so many times the nurse can wander the city centre looking for him. If she finds him, she buys him a coffee and tries to persuade him to stop smoking weed and to take his medication. Then she leaves and Nigel goes back to his chaotic paranoid existence. There are community support teams and services available to help people like Nigel, but when he is out of hospital he doesn't really have much interest in using them.

Nigel will always have a difficult, chaotic life, but it would be nice to think that we had the services available to keep him and everyone else safe. At the moment we don't. If he did take his medication regularly, he would probably stay fairly well. The problem is, like many people with mental illness, he just won't take it voluntarily. One option is to consider paying people like Nigel to take their antipsychotic drugs. It is a controversial idea but every time Nigel is admitted to hospital it costs the NHS thousands of pounds. If Nigel were paid £20 per month to come and get his injection of antipsychotic medication, it would probably be enough incentive for him to take it and he would almost certainly remain well. This would save thousands of pounds in hospital admissions and also reduce the harm caused to Nigel and those around him every time he becomes unwell. Many are against this idea, feeling that it degrades people with mental health problems. There are many stable, well-supported people with schizophrenia and other types of mental illness who take their medication readily without the need for financial incentives. Unfortunately, there are also an awful lot of Nigels.

Memories

I see about 40 patients a day and have been a doctor for several years. As you can imagine, over the years I have seen many thousands of patients. For the duration of their time with me, each patient has my full and undivided attention. But once they leave the room, my recollection of them fades quickly and they are filed into a grey blurry part of my memory somewhere between the names for the small bones in the hand and the West Ham team of 1985.

I'm sure many patients forget me as rapidly as I forget them, but I'm still surprised by the impression I can sometimes make as a doctor. I once got stopped in the post office by an elderly lady who greeted me as if I was her long-lost son. 'Dr Daniels! It is you, isn't it? It's me Rita, Rita Lloyd. You saw my husband Roger in A&E about four years ago.' I had absolutely no memory of her at all. Even digging deep into my brain, I pulled out Tony Cottee and Frank McAvennie (1980s West Ham legends) but no Rita and Roger Lloyd. 'You helped save my husband's life!' I was really racking my brain now. I should've recalled something. I endured many long and arduous shifts in A&E but it was rare that I ever helped save anyone's life. 'Roger had a tummy ache and everyone said it was just constipation but you examined him and said you thought there might be a more serious cause for the blockage. You sent him straight to the surgeons and they operated that night. He nearly died on the operating table but thankfully he pulled through.' 'Oh yes,' I said. I now had the names of nine West Ham players and two hand bones (although one of those might actually have been a foot bone) but still had no memory of Roger and his tummy pain. 'How is Roger doing now?' I asked. 'He died nine months later from the bowel cancer that was causing the blockage, but we are all so grateful for that extra time you helped to give us.' She gave me a big hug, shed a tear and left me to carry on in the post office. It's not often that I get a warm fuzzy feeling like that but it really was a vintage year for West Ham . . . and it's nice to think that I occasionally make a difference as a doctor.

Fighting

Tommy has a proper West country 'ooarr' accent that never fails to entertain me. He's not particularly blessed in the brains department and has a very high TTT score. TTT stands for tattoo to teeth. The rule is that if a patient comes in with more tattoos than teeth, they are probably going to have a fighting-related problem. This may seem like another unfair prejudice made by snobby middle-class doctors, but it is in fact a frighteningly accurate clinical sign.

''Allo, Doctor. I've come about my nose. It's sniffing, see. I can't sniffs on this side. And I can't sniffs on the other side, neither.' Tommy demonstrates with a long and unsuccessful attempt to breathe in through both nostrils in turn.

'See, Doctor – I can't sniffs nothing. I snores like a bear and I can't even smells my own farts.'

You didn't have to have a medical degree to spot the problem with Tommy's nose. It was clearly big to start with, but had unmistakably been broken on several occasions and now pointed in several directions at the same time. Judging from his multiple tattoos and missing teeth, I imagine that Tommy's nose has probably been punched out of shape, but it seems unfair to jump to conclusions.

'So, Tommy, it looks like you've broken your nose. Was that a sporting injury, perhaps?'

Tommy gives me a big toothless smile.

'No, Doctor. I broked it fighting. I broked it this way fighting in the pub and then my wife broked it the other way when we was rowing at home. Just the other day I think I might 'ave broked it again when I fell over pissed.'

I send Tommy off to the facial surgeons but warn him that they have quite a job on their hands.

I myself am pleased to say that I have never been hit. Although my nose is big, I am relieved that I have at least managed to keep it straight and I'm rather keen it remains that way. A recent report suggested that up to one-third of NHS staff have been physically assaulted at work. One of the reasons I have avoided violence during my years as a doctor is my natural tendency to exhibit cowardice at every possible opportunity. This was most clearly demonstrated when a fight broke out between two drunk patients one Friday night in the A&E department. When looking back at the CCTV footage with the police, several small nurses could be spotted bravely moving towards the action and attempting to break things up. Meanwhile, I could clearly be seen running away in the opposite direction towards the door.

I have been threatened on several occasions and it is easy to feel quite vulnerable when you are alone with an angry patient in a confined space such as an A&E cubicle or a GP surgery consultation room. People can get angry and aggressive when they are in pain or scared about their own health or the health of their loved one. Sometimes their aggression is part of an illness such as schizophrenia or dementia. Sometimes they are just drunken arseholes looking for a scrap. I have a simple rule. If someone is unnecessarily aggressive and abusive towards me, I won't see them. On one occasion in A&E a man was needlessly abusive and threatening towards one of the nurses. He was a little drunk but that was no excuse. He was shouting and swearing in front of young children and elderly people in the waiting room and, towards the end of a long and tiring shift, I decided that I was not going to put up with that sort of behaviour and I refused to see him. This made him more angry and he ended up kicking off big time and getting arrested. I could have probably resolved the situation peacefully by placating him verbally, making him a cup of tea and letting him jump the queue to be seen. But why should I?

When I made the decision not to see that man, I was in a busy A&E department with plenty of porters and a couple of burly security guys on hand to help protect me from getting a beating. Had I been less well protected, my cowardly instinct would have kicked in and I'd have happily treated him immediately as long I knew that it was going to prevent me ending up with a nose like Tommy's.

Class

After I call out my patient's name on the tannoy, it takes approximately 30 seconds for them to walk from the waiting room to my consulting room. In these 30 seconds I usually have a look at the patient's address and before they have even knocked on my door, I have already made many sweeping judgements about their health. I'm not proud of this as these assumptions are based purely on the street they live on. I know the local area well and, as with most towns, there are some streets with nice posh houses and others with small impoverished council flats. Class shouldn't play a part in how I treat my patients but it has such an effect on how people look after their own health, I can't help but consider it. This might simply sound like my middle-class prejudice but I promise you it isn't. Life expectancy for people in the lower social classes is significantly shorter than for those in the higher social classes and, in fact, even when you take out the risk factors of smoking, poor diet and obesity, simply being from a lower socioeconomic class independently increases the risk of having a heart attack.

From a personal perspective, I have worked in hugely different environments, from surgeries in inner city council estates to a surgery deep within the wealthy country lanes of the Home

Counties. The difference in the sort of health problems seen is extraordinary. Issues such as smoking, teenage pregnancy and obesity are three of the biggest health problems that the UK faces today, but although they get a lot of publicity, it is very seldom pointed out that they are principally conditions of the lower social classes. Of course, there are a few posh people who are overweight and smoke and even the odd rebellious private-school girl who gets pregnant, but ultimately these medical burdens are more related to a person's social environment than anything else. The onus is being put on to the NHS to solve these problems and, yes, we have a role to play, but ultimately if we could improve housing, education, attitudes and expectations, I think health would improve all on its own.

In most areas of our society, class is still extremely divisive. Our social class decides where we live, socialise, go on holiday and even where we buy our groceries. In many countries, private medicine ensures that class remains a divisive measure when it comes to the accessibility of healthcare. The NHS, however, means that the GP surgery is a bit of a melting pot for everyone. My waiting room can contain the posh ladies who lunch, sitting next to the homeless drug addicts who do crack. In theory, they should all get ten minutes of my time and have equal access to the NHS services available, but, of course, the reality is very different. Obviously, having private healthcare helps to oil the path to seeing the best doctors quickly, but even without paying, middle-class educated patients get a better deal. They ask more questions, are more demanding and are better able to access services available on the NHS. This has to go down as a failing on our part as doctors because we should be empowering our less-demanding and less-privileged patients with the information they need to get the best care available.

There are some wonderful GP surgeries in very poor parts of

the country and they do a fantastic job; however, some of the surgeries in poorer areas are run down and unloved, with unmotivated and unhappy staff. The surgery on a council estate I know of is an example of this. It is very busy because there are a lot of social problems on the estate and, as I've mentioned, social deprivation breeds medical problems. The staff have been threatened and the surgery keeps getting broken into, which doesn't help morale. Also there is the issue of money. I've talked previously about how GPs make money by hitting targets. This is a generalisation, but middle-class patients tend to be more active in managing and maintaining their own health than more socially deprived patients. This means that they are more compliant with medication and keeping appointments. Motivated healthy patients make it much easier for the GP to hit targets and, hence, earn money. The patients on council estates often have quite difficult, chaotic lives. If they miss their asthma review appointments or don't take their blood pressure medication, then this directly influences how much the doctors earn.

The reduced earnings of the council estate practice and low morale mean that it can't attract enthusiastic, dedicated new doctors. There is no shortage of GPs locally but the surgery on the council estate is currently being run by a series of locums. This is because one of the permanent doctors is on long-term sick leave with stress-related problems and, despite advertising, they can't find a GP to fill the other vacant post. The locum doctors never get to know the patients and as a result are generally fairly apathetic and disinterested. It is the patients who lose out. Middle-class patients would often demand improvements or move to a new surgery, but the patients on the estate often don't have the means to do this so put up with a poor service. It is yet another example of a two-tier health service. Nye Bevan must be turning in his grave.

Tingling ear syndrome

'I'm sorry, Paula, but I have absolutely no idea why your right ear has been tingling a bit since this morning. I don't think it is anything to worry about and it will probably go away on its own. Come back if it doesn't.'

I spend quite a lot of my time telling my patients that I don't really know what is wrong with them. This sometimes disappoints them terribly or at least makes them think that I'm a rubbish doctor, but the reality is that I see hundreds of patients with the odd ache or pain or tingle or discomfort and often I don't really know what is causing it. This isn't because I'm a rubbish doctor, it is just because we all get the odd funny ache or pain now and again and eventually it almost always goes away on its own. One of my colleagues tells his elderly patients that if they wake up one morning without any aches and pains, they have almost certainly died in the night! When I am faced with my patients' mysterious aches and pains, I am often tempted to make something up and prescribe a placebo, but gone are the days where we could completely bullshit our patients and get away with it.

My brother is not medical and went to the doctor recently

271

because one part of his arm was a bit red. His GP stroked his chin and then wisely stated that he thought my brother had a mild case of erythema. My brother was initially very impressed with this diagnosis. He didn't know what the word meant but it sounded like a convincingly rare skin disease. He then went home and Googled erythema only to find out that it means red skin. My brother had told his doctor that he had 'an area of red skin' and the doctor then cleverly diagnosed him with having 'an area of red skin'. Using a Latin word to make ourselves sound intelligent does work briefly, but the internet now means that our jargon can be rapidly exposed as the bullshit it really is.

Most aches and pains that I see get better on their own with a bit of time. Coming to see me tends not to make a great deal of difference to this. You might think I'm talking myself out of a job but I'm not. If a 20-year-old woman has a bit of a tingly ear from time to time, then I'll probably not know a cause or find a cure. However, a 60-year-old smoker with a tingly left arm might think his discomfort was equally trivial, but actually be having symptoms of a heart attack. This is where I come in. My job is to reassure the young person with a bit of a tingly ear but send the man with a tingly arm to hospital, as his heart might be about to stop.

If my healthy 20-year-old patient took her tingly ear and saw 100 doctors, healers or alternative therapists around the world, they would probably each come up with a different diagnosis. This is not because they are cleverer than me and know the real cause, but simply because they are being paid to give a diagnosis. If they can come up with a believable diagnosis, then they can sell a treatment. Telling someone that you don't know what is wrong with them and that they'll get better on their own is not a good way of making money if you work in a private health service. Fortunately for us, we have the NHS. GPs make money by jumping through hoops and reaching government targets, but not by making up diagnoses and then flogging you placebos.

Gary

I always found Gary to be slightly overbearing. He was a salesman of some sort and always shook my hand very firmly and maintained eye contact for a little too long. I was scared that one of these days he was going to talk me into buying a photocopier. This day he was a little more bashful.

'I need your help, Dr Daniels. I had a little mishap at the Christmas party with one of the girls in the office. It was just a bit of drunken fun, but she's just told me that she's got chlamydia. I'll be honest with you, Doctor, I'm fucking terrified. If my wife finds out, she'll leave me. I'm already on my last chance. We've got two kids.'

'Well, the best people to deal with this sort of thing are the doctors in the sexual health clinic. I could give you their telephone number.'

'I'm not going to the clap clinic, Doctor. If somebody sees me there, I'm a dead man. I've had a look on the internet and I just need some of this antibiotic called azithromycin. One tablet does the job and we can just sort this out here and now.'

'Well, it's not ideal. Really, it would be better to test you. Have you had any symptoms? Burning when you pee? Milky discharge from your penis?'

'I've had nothing like that but I'm not taking any chances and I'm not having you stick a swab down my little guy. I just need a prescription for the one-off antibiotic . . . and one for my wife.'

'Have you told her?'

'God, no! She'd leave me. Now this azithromycin stuff, would it dissolve in her tea? I was thinking about crumbling the tablet into a pasta sauce but was worried that the cooking process might damage it.'

'Look, I can't encourage you to be secretly drugging your wife with antibiotics. What if she has an allergic reaction? It's my name on the prescription. I would have to take responsibility.'

'Doctor, please work with me here. Man to man. My marriage is on the line. Why don't you prescribe me a double dose and what I do with the pills is my responsibility. I don't mind paying for them.'

'Look, I feel really uncomfortable about this. I appreciate your predicament but I'm not prepared to prescribe you this medication knowing that you're going to give some secretly to your wife.'

'Do you really want to be responsible for the break-up of a family, Dr Daniels?'

'To be fair, it wasn't me who cheated on my wife.'

'You're not paid to judge me, Doctor. Look, I've an idea. Why don't you call my wife in for a smear and while you're down there, you can do a quick swab for chlamydia.'

'Look, we can't just test people and give them medicines without them knowing. We need to have consent.'

'There must be something you can do. If you don't prescribe me these antibiotics, I'll get them off the internet and that's even more dodgy. God knows what I could be poisoning her with.'

'I've got an idea. Why don't you get yourself tested? It's only a urine test and then if you're negative, you don't have to worry.'

'And if I'm positive?'

'We'll cross that bridge when we get to it.'

Thankfully, Gary tested negative and I never had to worry about a second attempt by him trying to talk me into secretly drugging his wife.

Beach medicine

Last year I was lucky enough to have been lying on a white sandy beach with calm, crystal clear, blue waters lapping on the shore. It was a picture of idyllic tranquillity until a woman dropped down dead a few yards away. Had it been an episode of *Baywatch*, I would have run over heroically and, with sweat glistening on my tanned bulging biceps, I would have brought her back to life with a few seconds of mouth to mouth. The rescued lady would have been 22 years old with large false breasts and gleaming white teeth. After spitting out a couple of gulps of sea water, she would have gazed into my eyes with her make-up still perfect and declared her undying love for me.

Unfortunately, this wasn't an episode of *Baywatch*. The woman was a German tourist in her late seventies and was dead as dead could be. I did run over and try resuscitation and my wife bravely started mouth to mouth, which was impressive given that the German woman had vomited before collapsing. A crowd of onlookers developed and an ambulance was apparently on its way, but after 15 minutes of CPR, it became clear that this lady wasn't coming back. The problem we had now was what to do? The ambulance was coming from the other side of the island and could be another hour. The sun wasn't reflecting off my tanned rippling biceps because I don't actually have any. Instead, it was beating down on my pasty white back and I could feel that I was beginning to burn.

I really wanted to call it a day. Not just because I was getting sunburnt but because this woman was dead. In a hospital I would have 'called it'. This is where the team running the resuscitation makes a decision to stop. I am quite happy to make this decision in a hospital because I am surrounded by lots of other doctors and nurses and a hospital full of equipment. On this beach I had none of that. I didn't have a heart monitor to tell me if there was any electrical activity coming from the heart. I didn't have a blood glucose machine to tell me that she wasn't a diabetic with a very low blood sugar and I didn't have a team of other doctors to agree that it was the right decision. I did, however, have my common sense. It would take at least another 45 minutes for the ambulance to reach us and then another hour on bumpy roads to get her to a small, poorly equipped hospital with no intensive care department. The husband had told me that she had survived a heart attack earlier in the year and so it didn't take a diagnostic genius to work out that she had probably just had a second one after returning from an overenergetic swim.

I decided not to go with my common sense and instead we carried on with the chest compressions and mouth to mouth. This was not because I thought that there was any chance of this woman surviving, but because her distraught-looking husband needed to feel that absolutely everything that could be done was being done. The other concern was a legal one. Once you start a treatment, it can be a thorny matter about deciding to stop. I wasn't in the UK and from a litigious viewpoint, it was a much safer decision to carry on with the pointless CPR. I had a big crowd of onlookers now and they were every bit an audience as our performance was purely for show. The ambulancemen did eventually arrive but, to be honest, they were fairly useless. They didn't have much equipment and they couldn't intubate (put a tube into the lungs to help breathing). They didn't even have a defibrillator (machine to give the heart an electric shock). Instead, they scooped her up on a stretcher, plodded along the beach to the ambulance and drove her to the hospital, continuing to resuscitate in much the same ineffectual way as me.

That beach really was gorgeous and although in no hurry to die myself, I can't think of a more perfect place to expire. To drop down dead on golden white sands after a swim in crystal clear waters seems a rather nice way to go. If it were me, I wouldn't then want some sweaty pasty English bloke to spend an hour jumping up and down on my chest in front of a crowd of nosy onlookers.

Gifts

One of my female patients has begun visiting me twice a week. During our consultations, she pulls in her chair very close to me and strokes my leg. She always kisses me when she leaves and has taken to buying me presents despite my objections. During our last consultation, she attempted (unsuccessfully) to slip me an envelope full of cash.

Ethel is 93 and her behaviour is generally thought to be a bit 'batty' and 'comical' rather than anything more concerning. Were I a young female GP receiving this sort of attention from a male patient, everyone would be a bit more concerned, but given that Ethel isn't exactly threatening my personal safety or my marriage, her affections remain nothing more than a source of amusement to the receptionists and other doctors.

Generally speaking, receiving gifts from patients can be awkward. Sometimes patients simply want to say thank you for putting in that extra bit of effort, but I generally feel uncomfortable receiving gifts. I'm being paid very well to look after my patients and so shouldn't really expect an extra incentive such as a nice bottle of wine at Christmas to do my job. I feel especially bad if a patient who I know doesn't have much money buys me an expensive gift that they can't afford. Declining the gift can cause offence but it is a difficult area.

Sometimes gifts put an odd slant on the consultation. I received a very expensive bottle of champagne from one of my patients one Christmas. The bottle was very happily received (and consumed), although I was slightly surprised as the patient wasn't someone that I saw very regularly. Two weeks later I received a form to complete with regard to his entitlement to incapacity benefit payments. The patient had been on long-term sick benefits for a long time but I did question his genuine need to be signed off work. I filled in the form honestly but I wonder whether the bottle of bubbly was an attempt to be a bit of a softener.

One of my colleagues once got left the entirety of the contents of a patient's house in her will. He had a big dilemma as to whether he should accept this and, after much debate, eventually decided to sell her belongings and give the money to charity. After spending a long weekend trawling through her possessions, he ended up having to fork out £200 to have everything taken away by a house clearance company, as there was nothing of any value whatsoever. He wasn't best pleased.

I can't speak for other doctors, but personally if a patient ever wants to thank me, I would love a card or letter expressing this. As with us all, it is nice to be told that we are doing a good job sometimes, even if it is simply what we are being paid to do. I'm not that keen on wine and chocolates make me fat. Envelopes of cash are a bit dodgy and will get me struck off, so a card is just right.

Politics

I know very little about economics and, to be honest, I don't really understand exactly why interest rates go up and down. My main concern is how much my mortgage payments are each month. Fortunately for us, we have the Bank of England to make decisions about interest rates. It is an independent organisation, unrelated to the ambitions of individual political parties and politicians, which works to maintain the stability of the economy. I have no idea who the individual members of the bank committee are. I imagine them to be wise old men with white beards who sit at a round table somewhere, possibly in a bank vault or a castle. Wherever they work from, the important thing is that as a nation, we generally seem to trust that the decisions that they make are the right ones and ultimately for the benefit of us all. I'm relieved that politicians who know little about economics aren't allowed to make dangerous decisions such as slashing interest rates to win votes. Unfortunately, we are not so lucky with regard to decisions made about healthcare.

All the recent big policies with regard to the NHS appear to have been to win votes rather than actually improve the service that it provides. They have been made by politicians who have never worked in a medical setting and are fairly healthy so rarely use the NHS. They are policies targeted to impress the important voters. People who are genuinely vulnerable and unwell don't tend to vote and certainly don't swing elections. This means that the elderly and mentally ill are pretty much neglected. The worried well, however, are a much more important voting population. Young healthy commuters are the least wanting with regard to health require-ments, but the politicians need their votes. Opening surgeries on Saturday mornings, four-hour A&E waiting times and having choice over which hospital a GP refers you to are all examples of this. They are not necessarily bad ideas, but they have all been poorly thought through and instigated. Most of us who actually work in the health service could think of many more deserving causes to throw millions of pounds at.

My solution would be to have an equivalent of the Bank of England for the NHS: a small expert organisation that could basi-cally manage the NHS and help make the important decisions about how taxpayers' money is best spent on our health. It would be independent and not be affiliated to a political party or be directly affected by general elections. It could be made up of experienced nurses, hospital doctors, GPs, managers and patients who all have very recent and direct experience of being at the coalface of the NHS.

It may seem slightly undemocratic to have our NHS not directly managed by the elected government, but the elected politicians are clueless morons and keep fucking things up! Would it work? I don't know. Would it just add another tier of ineffectual managers? I hope not. Would it be worth a try? I think so.

Passing judgement

I know I can appear judgemental in my description of some of my patients. I don't mean to be. I try to treat all my patients equally and fairly. If I'm judgemental at times I think that it is not because I'm a doctor but simply because I'm human.

As a doctor, it can be difficult not to allow my own personal morals to reflect on how I view and treat a patient. For example, one morning I spent a long, tearful consultation with a lovely couple in their late thirties who had just failed in their fifth attempt at IVF. They had run out of money and hope and were emotionally distraught at the recognition that they would never conceive their own children. Later that morning, a woman came in requesting her fifth abortion. I don't have any ethical problem with abortions, but I did find myself judging her. Did she realise how hard it was for some people to conceive? Did she consider how much it cost the NHS each year to perform so many abortions? Contraception is free and readily available in this country. How could she have been so careless so many times?

I also found myself feeling very judgemental during a child protection case conference. I was in a meeting with social workers, health visitors and other professionals discussing what should be done with an unborn baby belonging to one of my patients.

I knew the mum-to-be well and, quite frankly, I thought she would make an absolutely terrible mother. She was rude, aggressive and always in trouble with the police. The dad wasn't on the scene and her own family had disowned her. I just didn't believe that she was the right person to give that baby the best start in life. Everyone in the meeting was very professional and positive. They were looking to implement extra support for the mum to help her with her new baby. I tried to be positive, too, and I do think kids are best off with their real parents, but a big part of me wanted to take that baby away at birth. I wanted to give him to the nice couple who kept failing with the IVF. I just felt that the child would have a better future with them than with its real mother.

Deep down I knew that I had no right to pass judgement on who would make better parents. I see my patients for ten minutes at a time and don't have the right to decide if someone should have their child taken away. What do I really know about parenting anyway? Would I like someone passing judgement on what sort of dad I am? Back at the case conference we all agreed that once born, the baby would be put on to the child protection register but stay with the mum and be closely monitored. I hoped I'd be proved wrong and that the new mum would do a great job. I know it is not my place to judge my patients but it can be very difficult sometimes.

The examination game

There is a lot of drama in medicine. As a doctor much of what I do is a performance rather than an attempt to actually gain important medical information. The examination is perhaps the most evident example of this. Examining patients is obviously important and sometimes I even find something abnormal . . . But a lot of the time the examination is a bit of a fraud. It is all part of my attempt to add mystique and importance to my job.

An example of this is when I visit one of my patients called Mr Briggs. Mr Briggs is well into his nineties and very frail. He has lots of things wrong with him, but unfortunately, they are mostly because of his excessive years and there isn't a great deal I can do about them. I'm fairly certain that Mr Briggs is going to die within the next year and my main objective is to make sure he remains as comfortable as possible and that I provide reassurance and support for him and his wife. Whenever I visit Mr Briggs, I check his blood pressure. I check it every visit and it doesn't change much. Even if it was raised, Mr Briggs has already said he doesn't want to start any new medication and certainly doesn't want to have any tests or investigations if he becomes more unwell.

Ultimately, I am not examining Mr Briggs for his physical health but for his emotional health. He is expecting me to examine him and by going through the motions, I am offering reassurance. Human-to-human contact is comforting. I am English so I don't give Mr Briggs a hug. Instead, I use a blood pressure cuff and a stethoscope to reach out and make some soothing physical contact with this dying man. 'Strong as an ox,' I often say after listening to his heart. It sounds patronising written here but I know that Mr and Mrs Briggs are reassured by my words. 'I wish the rest of my body was as strong as an ox,' Mr Briggs will reply as I shake his hand on leaving. Sometimes I wonder whether my examinations of Mr Briggs are actually as much for my benefit as for his. If I didn't have the extra gimmick of my stethoscope and blood pressure machine, how could I justify my visits? They are the instruments that define me as a doctor and without them I could simply be a visiting neighbour or the local vicar.

I am clearly not the only doctor who sometimes uses the examination as a bit of a show. One of my colleagues was visiting an elderly patient to give him a check-over and to reassure his wife. He had already mentioned that he would have a listen to his chest but then found that he had left his stethoscope at the surgery. Not wanting to admit this, he instead took out a 2p coin from his pocket and carefully placed it at various points on the patient's back. He was using the coin to mimic the bell of his stethoscope and as the patient was facing the other way, he imagined he would be none the wiser. Apparently, the patient seemed happy enough but just as my colleague was on his way out he stopped him: 'Just one thing, Doctor. I've seen some things in my time but I've never seen a doctor listen to my chest with a 2p coin.' The doctor hadn't noticed the mirror on the dresser that enabled the patient to watch him examining him. My colleague came clean and apparently they had a bit of a laugh about it. Just a lesson for us all not to ever try to pull the wool over our patients' eyes!

Sex

An astounding part of being a doctor is that a complete stranger can walk into my consulting room and within two minutes I can be asking them about their deepest, darkest sexual habits. A full sexual history is vital for accurately diagnosing and treating many illnesses. It is also a great way to find out exactly what people get up to behind closed doors! I am still amazed by my patients' sexual escapades and also about how honest, open and unembarrassed they are when telling me all about them. My patients make me feel very boring as they recall tales of dogging, rimming, fisting and various other sexual behaviours that I have to Google in order to know what they are talking about.

The youth in my area seem to be amazingly promiscuous and I was astonished when I met a patient who had kept her virginity until she got married at 23 years old. Her husband had apparently done the same and they had been using condoms for a couple of years until the previous month when they had decided to start trying for a baby. Jane, the woman in question, came to see me complaining of a creamy white vaginal discharge that she was now getting after sex. I feared the worst. I was sure her husband must have been having an affair and that she had caught some kind of sexually transmitted infection. I ordered a full set of vaginal swabs but everything came back as normal. It was only when she returned to see me and I asked her to explain her discharge symptoms in a little more detail that I realised that the post-coital discharge she was describing was actually just her husband's semen.

Money

Do GPs earn too much? That has certainly been the general consensus of the media over the last few years. I personally don't know any GPs who earn £250K as reported by the press; however, most GP partners who work full time earn over £100K, which seems a lot of money to me. I am not a partner myself but do fairly well out of being a locum GP and just a few years ago I was working considerably more hours as a hospital doctor for less than half the money.

The reason GPs earn so much is mainly political. I appreciate that many of you will be fairly uninterested in this and have bought the book to hear some amusing stories about patients coming in with unusual objects stuck up their bum, etc. If this is you, please skip to the next chapter.

In defence of our high earning:

We are highly trained – on average, it takes about 10–12 years to become a GP from starting medical school.

We have a stressful and difficult job.

We work hard. Most GPs work long days with lots of evening meetings and commitments.

We have a high tendency to be sued and pay £5,000 per year on our defence union fees.

We are generally very popular with our patients, with 9 out of 10 of you stating that you were very happy with the services provided by your local GP practice.

We provide a very efficient service. It has been quoted that it costs the British taxpayer about £20–25 for a visit to a GP. The value of this is very evident when compared to a visit to an A&E department, which costs £75 per attendance, and one visit to a walk-in centre costs £37. Amazingly, one visit to an out-patient department costs around £150.

The time spent per consultation with your GP has trebled since the NHS was created.

We earn peanuts compared to Premiership Footballers!

In criticism of our high earnings:

Our training is long but not as long as the training for hospital doctors, yet we tend to have higher earnings than most hospital consultants.

We do work hard but most GPs no longer have to see patients during weekends and nights, unlike most of our hospital colleagues.

We perform a vital role but so do hospital doctors, nurses, teachers, social workers and most of the public sector. Our pay is disproportionately higher.

Why do we earn so much?

We are only earning lots because we are reaching the targets the government sets us. The current GP contract was made by the Labour government, who foolishly didn't think we would achieve these targets. GP partners are generally bright, motivated people and when they realised that they could earn considerably more money by jumping through some hoops they quickly learnt to jump and became very good at it.

I've talked a bit about targets before. They are called Quality and Outcomes Framework (QOF) points and basically involve us fulfilling certain criteria with certain patients. For example, if I have a patient who has had a stroke, the practice earns points if his blood pressure is regularly checked and is well controlled. There are targets such as this for patients with asthma, diabetes, mental health problems, epilepsy and many more chronic conditions. Within a couple of years most surgeries worked out that they can actually reach these targets and make a lot of money. Technology has helped a lot and we now all have systems installed on our computers that flag up all our patients who need tests to reach our targets.

For example, every time a patient who has had a stroke walks in, the computer will flash up that his blood pressure is too high and will carry on nagging me until I have entered his reading on the computer. If the blood pressure is above a certain target level, it will nag me until I have given him enough blood pressure drugs for the target to have been reached. This is why sometimes you might come to see your doctor to grab some lotion for your child's head lice and the GP will check your blood pressure, ask if you smoke and get you to fill in a questionnaire about your mood. Your GP might not particularly care about any of these things and neither may you, but if we record this information on the computer, then we earn more points and more money.

It doesn't take long to do a blood pressure check or ask about smoking, but to reach some of the targets requires quite a lot of work. For example, if you are diabetic, there is a long, time-consuming list of data that needs to be input on the computer. This sort of information can't be quickly gathered in a normal consultation when you pitch up for something else. GP partners have realised this and much of the tedious data collection is best done by practice nurses. Paid considerably less than us, they do a lot of the work and basically earn the GPs their big salaries.

So if GPs are reaching all these targets and are earning all this money, why on earth did the government agree to the current GP contract? The main reason was that morale among GPs was at a particular low a few years ago. This was mostly because they were working long antisocial hours in difficult conditions without much reward. Lots of GPs were ready to retire early or move abroad and in some areas it was becoming impossible to fill GP posts. If it takes over ten years to train a GP, a shortfall could have led to a real crisis. A dearth of GPs would have meant patients waiting even longer for an appointment. Healthcare can be an election breaker and I think Labour probably felt that unless they did something to encourage GPs to stay in the profession, they could have lost the general election in 2005. The increased salary, together with the removal of an expectation that GPs would work evenings and weekends, prevented the early retirement of many very good GPs. It has also encouraged a large number of excellent young doctors to move into general practice when previously they might have chosen to stay in hospital medicine or move abroad. Many female doctors have been retained within the profession because there are now better options for family-friendly working hours. This has improved the quality of GPs and also meant that the crisis of a GP shortfall was avoided. Begrudgingly, I also have to admit that despite hating the tick-box culture, the targets are also likely to have contributed to generally better health promotion and chronic disease management.

The other aspect that needs to be remembered is that, although our wages are ultimately taken out of NHS coffers, GP surgeries are actually small, privately run businesses, making their own management decisions about pay, services, appointments and the day-to-day running of the practice. They do, of course, have to follow a huge number of regulations that are provided by the PCT and Whitehall, but they are still autonomous in many respects. As with all businesses, if the GP surgery works effectively and efficiently, it will earn more money. The practice will also get money if it branches out and provides new services such as minor surgery. The partners can then decide how that money is spent. They can choose to spend the money on improving the practice, or they can pocket the cash themselves. To be fair, most GPs have done a bit of both. Carrots are being dangled to GPs and for those who have the motivation and energy to set up new services and reach targets, the high wages are there for the taking.

Many of the extra services that can now be provided by GPs are being taken from hospitals. For example, the PCT might decide that they are paying too much money to the hospital to provide vasectomies. The hospital may have been providing vasectomies for years, but running any service from a hospital is expensive. The hospital is not interested in profit, so may well be running a fairly inefficient service. A GP might see the opportunity to undercut the hospital by training himself to do vasectomies and performing them at his surgery instead. He will then be slated in the press for earning loads of money, but by undercutting the hospital he will actually have saved the NHS considerably more than he earns. The GP is being well paid but has taken on a new responsibility and skill. He is also taking the risk that the service he is providing might be undercut by somebody else in the future.

This may all leave a slightly unsavoury taste in your mouth and I certainly didn't expect to have to get involved in the competitive cut-throat world of business when I chose to become a doctor. A few good GPs have rejected all of these modern changes and instead just do what they have been doing for years. They ignore targets and simply stick to trying to do the best they can for their patients. These are the GPs who don't earn as much money but have an honest wholesome glow about them. Good for them, but they are slowly being forced out of general practice as the brave new world order takes over.

As a young and sometimes still idealistic GP, I am trying to work out how to play the game. I want to make a good living but not let the greed and madness of medical politics engulf me. I will probably become a salaried GP. These doctors are employed by partnerships and earn a set wage for a set number of hours. They don't take a share of the windfalls acquired by meeting targets, but they do often do a lot of the work to reach those targets. They earn about £60–70K per year and avoid a lot of the bureaucracy and paperwork that the partners have to put up with.

Angela

One Saturday night I was working for the on-call GP service again. I was sitting in a small cold Portakabin in the main hospital car park and was covering the emergency GP calls for the entire town. I didn't know any of the people calling up but most of the problems could be dealt with over the phone and if not I could always drive round to do a home visit.

It was actually a fairly stress-free evening and after calls reassuring a couple of first-time mums and a brief visit to see an old lady with a urine infection, I was almost ready to go home. It was nearly 11 p.m. when the phone rang and I decided to take a last call:

Patient: May I ask who I'm speaking to?

Me: Certainly. My name is Dr Daniels. How can I help this evening?

Patient: Hello, Dr Daniels. My name is Angela and I'm going to kill myself right now and it's all your fault.

At this point the phone went dead. I tried to phone her back but the line was permanently engaged. The computer flagged up her telephone number and address but nothing else.

I had never met Angela before but apparently I was about to become responsible for her death. Even at my most narcissistic, I knew that I was unlikely to be important enough to single-handedly inspire the suicide of a complete stranger. I also very much doubted that Angela had any intention to actually die. The problem was what did I do now? I knew absolutely nothing about her. My gut instinct was that she was probably just a time-waster and the best thing to do would be to completely ignore her.

The problem was that the phone calls to the on-call doctors were recorded so if she was to be discovered dead tomorrow, I couldn't claim ignorance. The coroner's court case would be very embarrassing as I tried to explain why I did absolutely nothing after being told explicitly about a suicide attempt. 'I thought she was just a bit of a time-waster, your honour' probably wouldn't be a very successful line of defence.

Very reluctantly, I drove to the house. As I pulled up to her address there was already a pissed-off-looking ambulance crew at the scene. They had also received a phone call threatening suicide from Angela. Nobody was answering the door and after much pointless shouting through the letter box, we grudgingly decided we really needed to break in. One of the paramedics apologetic-ally told me that they weren't allowed to break the door down for health and safety reasons. I would have happily kicked the door down but was held back by general weediness. We made a contrite call to the police, who, after an hour or so, came round and with irritating ease bashed down the front door with one kick.

We all charged into the house and ran into each room in turn loudly shouting Angela's name. I dashed into the bathroom and then stopped dead. There was a woman lying in the bath. Her face was under the water with open eyes staring up at the ceiling. I could feel my heart pounding and was frozen to the spot. I assumed she was dead but then spotted a couple of bubbles coming out of her mouth. Her eyes had also moved from staring at the ceiling and were now looking straight at me. I grabbed her under the arms and pulled her up out of the water.

She was barely out of breath and looked me calmly in the face: 'Are you Dr Daniels? You owe me a new door.' Angela had clearly been patiently waiting for us to break the door down before sticking her head under the water.

She had evidently carefully planned the whole episode and was wearing a black swimming costume to protect her dignity for our anticipated dramatic entrance. She looked distinctly pleased with herself as she sat up in her bath with two paramedics, two policemen and me, all crammed into her tiny bathroom expectantly waiting for her next move.

I called the on-call psychiatrist.

'Oh, Angela. We all know her a bit too well. Has she pulled one of her stunts again?'

The psychiatrist was greatly amused by my account of the evening's entertainment. Apparently, she had made well over a hundred 'suicide' attempts and to date had never actually come close to causing herself any real harm. The professional viewpoint would be that Angela was a vulnerable person who struggled with effective communication and expressed her frustrations by making elaborate cries for help. One of the coppers on the scene was slightly less sympathetic and suggested that she was, in fact, a time-wasting piss artist who, after over a hundred failed suicide attempts, should have got a bit better at it by now. The psychiatrist had a chat with Angela on the phone and agreed to see her in clinic the following afternoon. I went home to bed.

I don't like some of my patients

Marcus Smythe is one of my patients and I just don't like him. He is privately educated and well-spoken but also has a drinking problem and beats up his wife. He is regularly rude and aggressive to the reception staff and bullies them into giving him immediate appointments that aren't necessary. He is also rude and demanding with me and if he doesn't get what he wants, he threatens to complain to his MP and write letters to the local paper. As each minute passes in his presence, my empathy, patience and tolerance rapidly dwindle away. During my medical school training, I learnt all about many rare diseases that I am unlikely to ever encounter, but I was never really given any preparation for how to deal with the Marcus Smythes of this world.

I love the fact that my job allows me to meet all types of people of all ages and backgrounds. It is the best part about being a doctor and of the several thousand patients I see each year, I'm rather fond of most. There are, however, one or two patients like Mr Smythe who regularly irritate and infuriate me. All doctors dislike one or two of their patients but, with the exception of occasional confessional whispers between close colleagues, we rarely admit to it. I had already been a doctor for several years when a consultant psychiatrist took me aside and told me that it was okay to dislike some of my patients. Hearing those words was like a huge weight being lifted off my shoulders. I was able to release my guilt that had been bubbling beneath the surface and eating away at me from the inside. It felt immensely liberating to now admit these feelings and reassure myself that they were normal and, in some ways, healthy. The revelation for me as a doctor was that while I now felt able to admit to myself my personal dislike of a patient, it must not stop me from treating him or her as fairly and professionally as I would any other patient.

Boundaries

Mark is about my age and I can't help but like the bloke. He is friendly, funny and interesting and if he wasn't one of my patients, I imagine he could well be one of my friends. He has bipolar disorder, which means that he can get very depressed at times and at others can become as high as a kite and dangerously manic. It is a tough condition to live with and I like to see him every few weeks to make sure everything is stable.

After a few months I've got to know him quite well. I know about his job and his family and his relationships. He can see the funny side of his illness and he makes me laugh with some of the stories he tells. Each time he comes to see me he asks how I am. Lots of my patients ask me this but most don't actually want me to answer. People visit the doctor to gratefully offload in one direction only. I don't have a problem with that, but Mark is different. We get on well and I genuinely feel that he does care how I am. It feels odd him calling me Dr Daniels rather than using my first name and I think that he would like me to take down my professional barrier and have our consultations as more like chats between two friends.

It is very tempting to give in and do just that. My days at work can be long and lonely. I am constantly speaking and interacting with people, but at the same time I'm not really allowed to be my real self or relax. I would love to have a proper chat with Mark and tell him a funny story about my weekend or let him know what really pissed me off about something that happened that morning, but I don't. I keep the barrier up for the protection of both of us. Mark is not my friend, he is my patient. If he viewed me as a friend, he might feel uneasy disclosing something to me. He might worry about what I thought or care about my opinion of him. At some time in the future he might become really unwell and need advice he doesn't want to hear, or worse still one day he might need sectioning. How could I act objectively as his doctor if I regarded him as a friend? It might come across as a bit stuffy calling myself Dr Daniels and refusing to talk about myself to patients, but boundaries are important. Mark has other friends but I'm his only GP. The doctor–patient relationship is unique and worth maintaining.

Smoking

Regardless of why a patient comes to see me, I am required to ask them if they smoke and if they say yes to give them 'smoking cessation advice'. I do this because it is probably a good idea that my smoking patients give up. I also do it because it earns the practice points and we all know what points mean.

Personally, I've never been that convinced about giving smoking cessation advice. I have tried various techniques and am not sure any of them really work. Here are a few of my best efforts:

'Smoking is bad for you' (patient probably knows this).

'Smoking will kill you' (patient probably knows this, too, and now I'll have put their blood pressure up, which will mess up my hypertension targets).

'Smoke if you want to, I really couldn't give a monkey's' (reverse psychology – maybe they'll give up to spite me).

'Stop smoking right now!' said in an authoritative paternal doctor-type way (patient would probably laugh because I'm not very good at being authoritative – ask my cat).

As with all addictions, beating them is only possible when the addict is really ready to give up, hence I only give smoking cessation advice when it is the patient's idea. Sometimes I'll give my smokers a bit of unsubtle prompting: 'Hmm, you've had a fair few chesty coughs this winter. Why do you think that is?' If the 40 per day smoker insists that it is because of an allergy to the neighbour's rabbit or the office's air-conditioning system, I don't bother with stop-smoking advice. If they recognise that smoking is harming them and genuinely want to give up, I am only too happy to give as much help, encouragement and nicotine patches as humanly possible.

Angry man

Angry man is red in the face and if I didn't know it was medically impossible, I wouldn't be surprised to see steam billowing out of his ears in a cartoon-like fashion.

'You need to give me some diazepam to calm me down, Doctor. I'm on edge. I feel like I'm going to hit someone!'

'Why are you so upset at the moment? Would you like to talk about it?'

'Look, Doctor, I'm not here to talk about my problems. I need you to give me something to calm me down.'

'I'm sorry but I don't prescribe diazepam for anger. We need to find a better way of dealing with the problem. I know of a very good anger-management course I could put you in touch with . . .'

I didn't think angry man could get any angrier, but I am wrong. He starts beating the desk and he pushes his face next to mine.

'Look, if you don't give me something to calm me down, I don't like to think what might happen. I could really fly off the handle and hurt someone. You could be responsible for someone really getting hurt.'

'If you hurt someone, you need to take responsibility for that yourself.'

Angry man stands up menacingly and, for a moment, I think he is going to hit me. I cower inwardly and wish my nose wasn't quite such a large target. Angry man calls me a fucking disgrace to the medical profession and then he leaves. I actually think that my complete lack of physical presence is a great advantage in these situations. I look about as menacing as an anorexic kitten playing with some cotton wool and this seems to deter even the most threatening of would-be nose breakers.

As the door slams, I give myself a few moments to compose myself and then carry on with the afternoon surgery. The rest of the day continues uneventfully and after Mrs Gibson's exceptionally large haemorrhoids and yet another 'funny turn' from Mr Polucovski, angry man's outburst is but a distant memory.

Two hours later I am standing at the checkout in Sainsburys, having stopped off on the way home from work. The boy on the checkout is particularly slow and I am regretting that I didn't pick the next queue over which seems to be travelling at twice the speed. The man behind me is putting his shopping on the belt and as I glance up, my heart skips a beat. It is angry man. We are trapped in the slowest checkout queue in history and the antagonism of our last meeting has switched to an overwhelming awkwardness. It is too late to swap to another till so we both shuffle along uncomfortably in the quiet confinement of the queue.

Earlier this afternoon I had imagined angry man to be in a perpetual state of rage, but now as my eyes browse over his shopping, I begin to see another side of him. I am relieved to see that he isn't buying a baseball bat and a book about serial killers. Instead, his basket holds a bunch of fair-trade bananas, some extra soft toilet paper and a Harry Potter book. Suddenly, angry man isn't the big scary man that he was a couple of hours ago. This opportune insight into the man behind the fury warms me to him slightly. I consider trying to find a few words to break the ice, but our super-slow checkout boy has finally managed to scan all my items and it is time for me to pay. As I leave, not-so-angry man gives me an awkward nod and I wonder if our next encounter in the surgery might be a little less heated.

Maintaining interest

After practising medicine for some time, the average grumpy doctor will have seen many thousands of patients pass before him or her. In the early part of our careers we greet every medical condition with genuine intrigue and gusto, but as the years pass it can become harder and harder to muster up the enthusiasm to keep ourselves awake during slow afternoon surgeries.

Having said that, there are a few ways in which you, the patient, can grab the attention of even the most indifferent of doctors:

1. *Have a rare condition.* Your diagnosis should be common enough that we learnt about it at medical school but rare enough to be something that we have never actually seen before in the flesh. Be warned, however, that if it is so rare that we can't recognise it or have never heard of it, our feelings of incompetence will lead to frustration and resentment, which will most likely be taken out on you.

2. *Have a diagnosis with a good name.* I love the way *molluscum contagiosum* rolls off the tongue. The delightful Latin words entertain me so much that I have forgiven the fact that the

condition they describe is an extremely mundane skin lesion that I have seen many hundreds of times.

3. *Make me laugh.* I will pardon a boring medical condition if it was obtained in a comical fashion. Sprained ankles are very dull but you will be entirely absolved if you managed to achieve your sprain by trying to do the moonwalk in a kebab shop while dressed as Scooby-Doo. If you actually just sprained your ankle by stepping awkwardly off the kerb, make up a more entertaining story and your doctor will view you in a better light.

4. *Be attractive.* When I was working in A&E, the orthopaedic surgeons were famous for avoiding seeing patients at any cost. The only time we ever saw them demonstrate any degree of enthusiasm about their chosen profession was when a particularly beautiful dance student injured her knee. I'm sure she didn't really need admitting but they insisted that they kept a close eye on her on the ward for a few days.

5. *Have a truly embarrassing problem.* It must be awful to have to tell your doctor that you have an object stuck up your bottom, but if it is any consolation, it will absolutely make your doctor's day. For me, the icing on the cake is always the ridiculous accompanying explanation: 'So I was trying to save water by washing the vegetables while also taking a shower and then I slipped and what are the chances of landing on that courgette . . .'

I am proud to say that I do listen and show interest in my patients because I still maintain enthusiasm for my job. This is not because my day-to-day work in general practice is on the cutting edge of medical science, but because I have a genuine interest in the people and the stories behind the science of the illnesses.

Of course, quite rightly when you are ill or injured, you have absolutely no reason to give two monkeys' whether your condition holds any academic curiosity or entertainment value to the doctor you're seeing – and why should you? Just one thing, though, if at the end of a long surgery you are 15 minutes through a monologue describing the detailed chronology of your athlete's foot, don't be overly offended if your doctor's eyes glaze over somewhat.

The future?

If you get a bunch of GPs in a room together, it won't be long before they start moaning about their jobs. This never ceases to amaze me, as I think we have it fairly good at the moment. We are paid well, work good hours and have an interesting and rewarding occupation. Despite this, GPs spend a great deal of time complaining about almost everything. I even heard a couple of GP partners complaining about how high their tax bill was going to be this year. I couldn't help but point out that if they were going to earn 120K, then they couldn't really expect any sympathy for paying a bit more to the treasury come April!

Some of my older patients reminisce fondly about the time when their own GP was on call 24 hours a day and was always on hand for an emergency visit. My uncle was one of those GPs. He would disappear from family dinners to deliver a baby, get home at 5 a.m. and then start morning surgery at 8 a.m. with a huge line of patients queuing out into the street. There is a wonderfully romantic, old-fashioned idea about that bygone time of the loyal and dedicated family GP. My auntie still has her late husband's ex-patients stopping her in the street and telling her what a wonderful doctor he was. My uncle had no life outside of his work and rarely spent any time with his family. He missed his children growing up and dropped down dead shortly after retiring. I wouldn't want to have had his life. My generation of young GPs is mostly much better at finding a balance between work and home life. I'm sorry that my patients have to see a GP they don't know if they need a doctor on a Sunday night or while I'm on holiday, but I have a life too.

All in all, I'm quite positive about the future of general practice. There are always scaremongering stories about big supermarket chains setting up surgeries and shipping in lots of Eastern European doctors to take over our jobs. I think this is unlikely. Yes, patients grumble about struggling to get through on the phone or their doctor running late, but individually most GPs are quite well liked and valued by their patients. My experience of patients is that they are a fairly loyal bunch. I'm not sure that a huge number would be lured away to Tesco if they opened surgeries at the back of their stores. I can see that some would be attracted by the convenience of supermarket doctors, especially if they ran a 24-hour service, but ultimately most patients like the familiarity and friendliness of their local practices. Although there is a lot of potential profit to be made out of running GP surgeries, there is also a hell of a lot of red tape and hoops to jump through. I'm not sure whether Tesco would really want the bother. I may eat my words someday but I think that our jobs and future are fairly secure.

Tariq

I found my first few consultations with Tariq frustrating. I struggled to understand his English and he never seemed to have much physically wrong with him. The consultations were always a bit disjointed and he always seemed reluctant to leave. Another wasted consultation, I would think to myself as he finally left my room.

Gradually, after his first few visits, Tariq began to open up to me. He was in his mid-twenties and had been tortured in a Sudanese jail after being arrested for political activity at his university. He had arrived here hidden in a lorry and was currently seeking asylum. He lived in a homeless hostel with mostly alcoholics and heroin addicts and spent his days aimlessly wandering the streets of the town centre. He was the sort of person I might walk past every day without noticing, but behind the sad tired face was a brilliant mind and a man desperate to work, study and make the most out of his life. Unfortunately, because of his asylum-seeking status, he was not entitled to do any of this. Instead, he looked enviously at the alcoholics and junkies that he lived with, knowing that as British citizens, if they so wished they could work, study and do many things that he was not entitled to do. Despite being understandably miserable here, Tariq was terrified that he would be tortured and killed if he returned to the Sudan, so he was stuck between an unpleasant rock and a horrifying hard place.

After his third or fourth visit, Tariq confessed to me that in the space of a whole week I was the only person he spoke to. If I wasn't a GP, I would not believe that in a busy cosmopolitan city a man could spend weeks passing the time without conversing with a single soul. Most people avoid seeing their doctor if they possibly can, but for Tariq, I was his only outlet to the rest of the world. I was the only person to whom he could talk about his feelings or even make small talk about the weather. In between my consultations with Tariq I spoke to many hundreds of people. I talked to work colleagues, friends and family, even the monosyllabic blokes I play football with. Tariq talked to no one. This must be torture for an intelligent, articulate and sociable young man.

In the soap opera that was Tariq's life, I was not just a walk-on part or an insignificant extra. For Tariq, I was the only other character in this episode of his life and was really quite important to him. Tariq had absolutely nothing physically wrong with him, yet my role as his doctor was vital and unique. He trusted me and I listened to his problems. He confided in me awful things that happened to him in his past and, more mundanely, I helped him fill out forms to aid his housing and finances. Helping Tariq wasn't putting my medical degree and years of training to great use, but my title as doctor and the ability of the NHS to make me available free of charge enabled me to reach out to another human and make a huge difference to his life. I have stopped grumbling that I'm overqualified to help someone fill in a form and instead appreciate the honour and privilege it is to be able to call myself a doctor working in the front line for the NHS.

Babies

It was my first night as a medical student on the delivery suite and I was excited at the prospect of helping to bring a new life into the world. To my horror, the first baby I saw was the life-less body of a stillborn. I had stayed away from the traumatic birth but the whole unit could hear the dead infant's mother wailing in grief as she pushed out her stillborn child. The midwife asked me to keep her company as she cleaned and dressed the body before it was taken down to the morgue. I can still clearly remember looking down at him. His features were perfect but his lips were almost completely black and the rest of his body a shade of dark purple. He had never had the chance to breathe in oxygen and turn pink. The pregnancy had apparently been normal and the baby was a healthy size. Mum was two weeks past her due date and as she and Dad eagerly anticipated the onset of labour, their baby just stopped moving. A scan confirmed that the heart was no longer beating. The devastated mum went into labour knowing that her son had already died.

Ten years later I was holding the hand of my wife, nervously waiting for the birth of our first child. It was one of those times that I wished I wasn't a doctor. I could not get the awful memory of that dead baby out of my mind. The other dads-to-be in my antenatal class had different concerns. Mick, a plumber, was worried about his mother-in-law coming to stay. Matthew worked in advertising and was fretting about the financial implications of dropping to just one income. My only anxiety was that my baby was going to be born dead. I didn't share this with the group, or even with my wife, but it dominated my thoughts for the last three months of my wife's pregnancy.

It would appear that I'm not the only doctor who has been affected by what they have witnessed in obstetrics. The number of female GPs and obstetricians who choose to have Caesarean sections rather than natural births is much higher than in the general population. Doctors also tend not to allow themselves to go too far overdue before having labour induced. It isn't so much that medics know more than everyone else, it is just that we have seen more than anyone else. Doctors deal with the births that go wrong. Thankfully, these are a tiny minority but anyone who has witnessed a really traumatic birth can't help but be affected by the memory when embarking on that journey them-selves. When my newly born son gasped his first breath, I was awash with joy, but far more powerful was an overwhelming sense of relief.

During the first few weeks of his life, the enormous responsi-bility of being a parent dawned on me. What sort of person was this baby going to become? What could I do to give him the best chance in life? If I was a rubbish parent, would he grow up to be like some of my chaotic and troubled patients? During my working day, I see an unfeasible amount of human suffering in one form or another. As I looked down on my innocent son, I wondered if I could really protect him from all that. What if one day he told me that he wanted to be a doctor? Would I try to put him off? In spite of everything, I love my job and have no regrets. I'd turn to him and say: 'Go for it, Son! Being a doctor is an honour and the greatest vocation there is.' However, if I had the slightest inkling that he could be a professional footballer and one day play for West Ham . . .

Read on for some brand-new chapters from
Dr Daniels . . .

Why do people get sick?

There was a tabloid article recently about a woman who lived to 103 years old and apparently she put her longevity down to never having had sex. Now this is clearly simply a silly tabloid article not meant to be taken too seriously, but it does illustrate the tendency we have to believe that things are as they are for a reason. Whether it is good health or illness, we seem to need to be able to explain it in terms of cause and affect in order to provide some meaning in our lives.

As a GP, I find this happens a lot to my patients as they try to rationalise the things that are happening to their bodies. For those of us lucky enough to take our health for granted, it can come as quite a shock when something goes wrong. This is where someone like me comes in. On a good day I'll often be able to answer the 'What is it?' question and even sometimes help with the 'What can I do about it?' dilemma. But 'Why has it happened to me?' is usually the hardest question and I rarely offer a satisfactory response.

Religious patients will happily explain everything as an 'Act of God', but for those without strong spiritual beliefs, the search for meaning in their illness can be a lot more difficult to find. Sometimes our physical ailments clearly reflect how we have treated our bodies. We can't dismiss the significance of diet, alcohol, smoking and stress, but although this may help explain the pre-Christmas migraine or even the lung cancer in the 40-a-day smoker, it offers no answers to the parents of a child who has just been diagnosed with leukaemia.

Some of my more new-age patients explain cancer and other severe illnesses with talk of negative energies and suppressed toxic emotions causing disease. No GP would argue that our emotional and physical health aren't strongly linked, but to claim 'suppressed emotions' to be the sole influence on an illness as complex as cancer is offensive to all the good people who have suffered from it. Receiving a diagnosis of cancer is hard enough to deal with, without the unpleasant and bogus idea that someone's suppressed psyche is in some way to blame.

My explanation for the majority of the illnesses I see is much duller. The causes of most medical problems are multiple. You might have a bit of arthritis in your knee for several reasons; you're getting on a bit, you're a bit overweight, it runs in your family but most importantly you've got a bad knee because shit happens. It's not God's will or bad energies, it's just life and part of being a human. You're probably reading this and understandably questioning my bedside manner. To the real people who come to me with genuine pains and fears, I promise that I offer more empathetic words than those I have just written. I do however stand by my belief that excessive ruminations and introversion about causes for illness are mostly unhelpful. They are completely understandable, yet a mostly pointless attempt to find meaning when unfortunately there is none.

I have one patient who has had decades of problems with his sinuses for which years of investigations, medications and operations have offered little relief. Every time he comes to see me he has desperately searched for and then unearthed a new possible explanation for his symptoms. These have ranged from radiation by mobile phone receivers, to his sexual promiscuity as a teenager 40 years earlier. Each time, he wants my opinion on his latest theory and each time I shrug, curse the internet and admit that the reason for his chronic nasal discharge is a medical mystery for which I can offer no solution. I could spout some jargon about him having a genetic predisposition to excessive histamine release in the nasal mucosa, but although this might be closer to a cause than his teenage sluttiness or mobile phone radiation poisoning, it still doesn't really explain why his genes code for overly-excited nasal mucosa and mine don't.

For a few of my patients I do believe there is an exact and clear explanation for their symptoms but sometimes it can be a difficult place to go. One of my patients found her mum dead from a heroin overdose at the age of nine. She is 25 now and suffers daily from a large array of unpleasant emotional and physical symptoms. I'm fairly convinced that the vast majority of these stem from the psychological consequences of her childhood trauma, accompanied by the generally awful parenting that came before and after. When she recently asked me 'Why do I keep getting all these headaches, Doctor?' I bravely suggested that there might be a link between her childhood suffering and her current physical symptoms. Despite my attempt to propose this connection with tact and kindness, she stormed out of my room in tears, accusing me of disbelieving her physical complaints and demanding yet another brain scan. It would have been much easier to have just blamed mobile phone receivers.

Malcolm

Malcolm drank too much and his wife left him, so he drank some more and lost his job, then he drank some more and now he can't pay his rent and is being evicted. He never visits the doctor but today he sits before me clutching a letter from the housing department at the council. There is about one available council flat for every 100 applications in my city. Single men like Malcolm come pretty low on the priority list, so some young housing officer has written me a letter advising that he might be pushed up in priority if I could write a letter saying that Malcolm's mental state would be adversely affected by being made homeless.

I find this really irritating. Malcolm should be given a roof over his head, but does it need a doctor to say that his mental health would be affected by him being made homeless? Being made homeless must be an absolutely awful experience. Who wouldn't become depressed and anxious as a result? It feels to me like another attempt to medicalise a social problem. Malcolm needs some social support and help with his alcohol addiction. He doesn't need a patronising letter from me giving a medical diagnosis to his understandably miserable predicament. The sad thing is that even if I write a long and convincing letter, Malcolm will at best be moved up from low to medium priority, which in real terms still means that the council isn't going to give him his own flat.

At 7.30 that evening I get round to starting Malcolm's letter. The housing department at the council are going to pay me £25 for this pointless letter, which is money that I assume actually comes out of your council tax. I don't really want the £25 and I would happily exchange it for being home in time for my son's bedtime, which I am now going to miss. There is a homeless man right now bedding down in the doorway of our surgery. Wouldn't it be great if the council paid him the £25 to write the letter instead?

It might go something like this.

Dear council,

Living on the streets is really shit. It is cold and lonely and I often get beaten up. People generally ignore me, only occasionally offering a look of contempt. One time a pissed-up city boy thought it would be funny to urinate on me whilst I was sleeping. Would you feel depressed and anxious if this happened to you?

Yours sincerely,

A homeless bloke sleeping in the doorway of the doctor's surgery

A pair of glasses

I can get a bit grumpy at times, but I'm not generally a shout-down-the-telephone sort of bloke. Today was an exception and I found myself shouting down the telephone about a pair of spectacles. The woman sitting in front of me had been the victim of some really quite horrific domestic violence. She had been physically, sexually and emotionally abused for years at the hands of her husband, but when her two-year-old daughter started being beaten as well she bravely stood up for herself and fought back. The ensuing thrashing resulted in her neighbours calling 999 and to the credit of the police, social services and the council, her husband was charged with assault and she and her daughter were given emergency accommodation.

Mrs Abbasi was bruised and tearful but for the first time in her married life she felt safe. Her main problem this morning was that she couldn't see. Her husband had broken her glasses and she had no idea of how to get herself another pair. She is from Iran and her English was limited. Her husband had prevented her from taking English lessons and she was very much alone and penniless in a foreign country.

We had a long chat via an interpreter and I wondered whether she might be best off heading back home. She looked at me sadly and told me that as a single woman in Iran she was powerless. Her husband had every right to take her and her daughter back to his house and she would have absolutely no protection against his abuse. The law in Iran would always work in his favour and she could both lose her daughter and end up on the streets. Although England was a foreign environment for her and she literally had nothing to call her own, she did at least have the protection of the state and the ability for her and her daughter to stay safe. For this she was incredibly grateful.

There wasn't a great deal I could do medically for Mrs Abbasi that day, but after documenting her bruises and injuries in the medical notes, I explained that she was entitled to a free pair of glasses on the NHS. She looked extremely surprised by this prospect and it was the second time that I found myself thinking that perhaps the UK wasn't so bad after all. I called up our local opticians and explained that I was sending Mrs Abbasi their way for a free eye test and a pair of glasses. This is where the disagreement started. The manager of the opticians explained that without the correct paperwork from the benefits agency she couldn't be given the glasses. Mrs Abbasi didn't have any paperwork, and to return to her husband's flat would risk another life-threatening beating. I started getting angry. This poor woman was practically blind without her glasses and was trying to care for her two-year-old daughter. She didn't have a pot to piss in and all she needed was a cheap pair of specs. I don't often make a significant difference to one of my patients' lives during an average day in general practice, but this pair of glasses was my big chance. I wasn't going to let this jobsworth on the other end of the line prevent me. I started raising my voice and eventually the manager backed down and conceded that she would make an exception. The next day Mrs Abbasi came back in to see me, proudly sporting a pair of very unfashionable but sight-returning NHS specs.

A few months later, and Mrs Abbasi is now learning English fast and her daughter is thriving. She has been granted leave to remain in the UK and is starting a new life for herself. It makes me feel very proud to think that as a country we were able to offer her and her daughter that safety and security. From a personal viewpoint, I'm proud that despite knowing bugger all about ophthalmology, with a bit of phone shouting I was able to help someone to see again!

Stewart

Stewart was a big burly Scottish guy with an accent as broad as his gut. He had been summoned in by our targets manager to discuss his health. In other words he was messing up our QOF figures as his blood pressure and cholesterol were sky high and he wasn't taking any of his medication.

I decide that the softly softly method I've tried in the past won't work on Stewart, so I opt to go for the 'scare him into submission' approach.

'Stewart, you're like a ticking time bomb. You're only 63 but you have every risk factor for a stroke or heart attack possible. My computer has worked out that you have a 50 per cent chance of having one or the other in the next 10 years. You really need to stop smoking, lose some weight and take some tablets to control your blood pressure.'

I don't get the response I was hoping for.

'You're telling me that after everything that I've done to my body, I still have a 50 per cent chance of living for another 10 years? Bloody hell, that's a fucking medical miracle that is. Not one male member of my family has ever lived past 60, so I'm already one of life's winners, Dr Daniels.'

Stewart sits back in his chair with his arms crossed, looking rather pleased with himself as he continues.

'I'm fed up with all this "don't smoke, don't eat chips" nonsense I keep hearing about. I rather like the prospect of being a ticking time bomb. I've always wanted to go out with a bang and I'm hoping to "go off" at the ciggies counter at ASDA – can you imagine the mess when this little baby blows?' He says, proudly patting his hefty beer gut.

'Every man in my family has dropped down dead with a heart attack in his prime. Most of them have departed this life in the pub with a pint in one hand, a ciggie in the other and a smile on their face. Every woman in our family has dragged on into old age, seeing out their days soiling their knickers as a dribbling vegetable in an old folks' home. Are you really asking me to take those pills and give up my pleasures in life for that?'

I'm left rather speechless at that little homily. Realising that he was on a roll, Stewart decides to try and finish me off whilst I'm down.

'My next door neighbour took all those blood pressure and cholesterol pills that you doctors love prescribing. He never drank or smoked and was always at the gym and eating salads. Smug bastard he was, forever lecturing me over the fence about my health. Dropped down dead at 47 with a heart attack. Closer to your age than mine, he was. Ha ha ha ha – shouldn't laugh but I did smile when I heard the news.'

On that note, Stewart got up and went to leave.

'Just one more thing, Doctor, it gives me great pleasure to be messing up all your targets!!!! I hope it costs you loads of money. Ha ha ha ha.'

NHS reforms

I've signed up to represent my practice within my local GP consortium and as a dedicated believer in the ideals of the NHS, I can't help but feel like a traitor. When my child sits on my knee in years to come and says, 'Daddy, what did you do during the privatisation of the NHS?' what will I say? I've been told that we have no choice but to collaborate and join a consortium, but will I really have to admit that during the NHS's darkest hour, instead of fighting them on the beaches, I was one of Andrew Lansley's evil henchmen?

The reason GPs may start opting to commission private services is typified by our local NHS physiotherapy service. In short, it's rubbish. I saw a self-employed decorator this morning with shoulder pain. He is off work and would really benefit from some help to improve his mobility. It would probably reduce the number of painkillers he is taking and also might get him back to work quicker. He needs some physiotherapy now but he'll probably be waiting at least four months for his appointment. When waiting times are so long, appointments are often forgotten and missed. In fact I am fairly sure that right now the much-in-demand physios are spending half of their time sitting around twiddling their thumbs, due to such a large proportion of their patients failing to turn up. It's a ridiculous and inefficient system and it wouldn't function in the private sector, for obvious reasons.

The government have clearly looked at this and decided that the answer is to bring in independent companies who can compete to offer a better service, for less money and with shorter waiting times. If a private company in our town pitched a superior physiotherapy service in both quality and price, it would be very difficult for me and fellow GPs within the local consortium to try and stay loyal to our local NHS service. If we were to give the tender out to an independent provider we would be effectively privatising a service previously provided by the NHS. Once this begins, it will inevitably lead to a frightening progression that would be very hard to reverse, even with future changes in government.

Most GPs are against or at least very dubious about the NHS Bill which is going through parliament at the moment, but please don't think that this means that we are against change. It is impossible to ignore some of the obvious inefficiencies within the NHS and the frustrations and poor services that our patients are often subjected to. Does this then mean that currently struggling NHS services should be automatically taken over by a privately-run company? Would it not be simpler and cheaper just to make our local NHS services a bit better? Do we really have to introduce capitalism, market forces and competition to make this happen? Individually our local physios are very well trained and professional and my patients who do eventually get appointments with them tell me that they are wonderful. Improvement shouldn't need targets passed down from Whitehall or teams of management consultants on £150 per hour. It would simply need someone locally with a bit of clout and management experience to come in and kick the service up the arse.

Added to this is the frightening prospect of the private care providers going bust and then leaving patients completely in the lurch. This is illustrated by the financial difficulties faced by the company Southern Cross who ran many hundreds of private care homes. There was a real possibility that their vulnerable and elderly residents (customers) would have been made effectively homeless when the business went under.

We could definitely improve elements of the NHS by incorporating some pointers from the private sector, but personally I wouldn't include the 'making profit for shareholders' part. We need to be a bit more ruthless about bringing in change from within and although change is hard, and it is horrible for people to lose their jobs, there can be no excuse for the huge number of inefficient pen pushers and managers who seem to offer no benefit at all for patients or front line staff. As a GP, I am unexpectedly finding myself standing right at the centre of a historical crossroads for the NHS. Whilst accepting the need for change, I hope we don't automatically opt for spineless, uncritical collaboration. Perhaps we have it in us to do some fighting on the beaches after all.

Barry

Barry wants a medical report to support his compensation claim against the council. He tripped over on a loose paving stone and broke a rib. The 'no win no fee' lawyer reckons he's due a big payout and unfortunately, he may be right. The unusual aspect about the fall that caused Barry's broken rib was that it would appear he was actually on the way to the pub rather than on the way home. Falling over is something Barry does a lot of, although only at the frequency you might expect of someone who drinks ten pints of beer per day.

As I skim through his notes I can see that in the last two years Barry has had over ten A&E admissions. Each has required an ambulance call out and some degree of A&E input. They have all been either alcohol or smoking related, with several drunken falls and a few chest infections related to his smoke-damaged lungs. He had one operation to fix a broken wrist and on another occasion had to be stitched up after falling on some broken glass. There have been numerous other drunken injuries and two or three admissions for simply being overwhelmingly pissed. It is impossible to calculate the exact monetary costs of these admissions but the ambulance call outs, X-rays, operations, medications prescribed and staff costs must run into thousands. This is simply the cost that Barry's drinking and smoking has made to the hospital and ambulance service. The cost of the inhalers I prescribe for his emphysema cost over £1,000 per year and over the years his drinking has cost even more money in terms of the prison service, probation service and for the last five years, incapacity benefit (Barry is mostly too drunk to work). Less expensive, but perhaps more significant, are the missed appointments at the alcohol clinic. There is help available for Barry but he has consistently turned it down.

I grew up with the belief that a good society is one that looks after its sickest, poorest and most vulnerable members. I still believe this to be true, and during my naïve and idealistic teenage years I would relay this as the reason I chose to become a doctor. But Barry and a huge number of people I see every day in my surgery do test this belief. Barry could bring out the right-winger in the best of us, but despite my annoyance, I realise that he doesn't change my deep-seated support for a health service that is free to everyone at the point of delivery, and a social care system that helps keep people off the street and out of jail. I don't see how denying services or charging the likes of Barry would either change his behaviour or cost the state any less in the long term.

So if I believe Barry is entitled to free care, why does he make me feel so angry? What do I want from him? Well, I suppose a good start would be some gratitude! I want him to step back and realise how much he is given by the state. I want him to appreciate that when he falls down due to his own drunken stupidity, someone picks him up, takes him to hospital and puts him back together again. I want him to grasp that this all costs money and that it is principally paid for by all the hard-working people around him who pay their taxes. I don't want him to see his unfortunate fall on the way to the pub as a way of gaining a couple of grand out of our council tax payments that might otherwise be spent on schools or housing.

This morning Barry is in a rare state of sobriety, so I carefully explain the implications of his alcohol and smoking addictions on his own health and the financial health of the nation. I even talk about how skint the NHS is and how we all need to do our bit. He listens intently and then we share a thoughtful silence for a few moments. 'So when will that medical report be ready for me, Doc? I'm gonna take this council to the cleaners.'

Tuition fees

Of all the students to be hit with rising tuition fees over the coming years, student doctors will probably receive the least sympathy. Studying for five or six years, medical students will end up with larger debts than most, but unlike the majority of graduates we are almost certainly guaranteed a well-paid recession-proof job for life, with the added factor that our salaries principally come out of the public purse. The £45,000 in tuition fees that tomorrow's doctors might end up owing is also minimal in comparison to the actual cost to the taxpayer of putting us through medical school, which is probably more like £250,000 per doctor trained.

For many of the people that I went to medical school with, £9,000 per year tuition fees will be considerably less than the private school fees that were paid by their parents for the earlier part of their education. Medical school is still a fairly elite aspiration and although not many of us wear bow ties and go hunting at the weekend any more, as a profession, we still don't really represent the population that we serve.

The coalition government would argue that the change in tuition fees will enable more disadvantaged students to get into medical school, but the truth is this seems unlikely. When I started medical school in 1996 there were no tuition fees, but there was also a distinct lack of anyone who could be considered to be from a disadvantaged background on my course. For a state school boy, even a middle-class one like me, medical school was a massive eye opener to the world of the privileged. Culturally, it was an extension of public school with cricket club dinners, summer balls and rugby boys drinking each other's vomit.

I'm no sociologist, but the lack of working-class kids becoming doctors is fairly understandable when you consider the huge number of hoops that have to be jumped through in order to successfully gain entry to medical school. Not only do you need to get top A-level results, but you must be able to pad out your application with tales of work experience, charity do-gooding, sporting prowess and musical genius. You then have to be adequately well-spoken to impress during the medical school interview. With around 10 applicants for every place, the average 17-year-old entering this process profits greatly from the help and support offered by the winning combination of an elite school and pushy middle-class parents. Successful applicants have often benefited from expensive interview preparation courses, work experience provided by medical relatives or family friends, excellent references and word-perfect personal statements that have been carefully edited by well-practised tutors.

Interestingly, the one group of medical students who seem to be bucking the trend with regard to social class is the mature student cohort. Katie, the final year medical student I am supervising at the moment, is 29 and a single mum. She grew up in a very normal working-class household and rather than spending her mid teens cramming for chemistry exams and having piano lessons, she had perhaps a more typical adolescence spent bunking off school and drinking cider in the park. An unplanned pregnancy, shotgun wedding and then a short and unsuccessful marriage meant she had to grow up quickly. With the help of her parents who provided childcare, Katie then decided to study for a psychology degree. After belatedly realising her true potential, she took the big step of applying to medical school. Katie is by far the best medical student I've ever taught. She is bright and learns quickly, but most importantly she has a fantastic bedside manner and her ability to put patients at ease appears effortless. She is the sort of person you meet and think 'I wish you were my doctor!' Katie and her family are making a massive sacrifice for her to study medicine. As a mature student who already has a degree, were she to be starting medical school in 2012, she would almost certainly have to pay her tuition fees up front, regardless of her low household income. Even just finding the £9,000 to cover her first year would make studying medicine an absolute impossibility for her.

I'm not suggesting that a person's social class has any bearing on his or her ability to be a good doctor, but when the NHS is all about delivering universal health care, it seems a shame that the medical profession seems so resistant to breaking through class boundaries within its own ranks. The extra life experience and more varied social backgrounds that mature medical students bring to our profession are refreshing. Although there is no guarantee that these mature students will automatically make better doctors, their worldlier outlook on life has to be a positive for UK medicine and should be encouraged. I really hope that the potential financial barrier created by the forthcoming increase in tuition fees doesn't close the door in their faces.

Please don't outsource our receptionists

There has been talk for some time about far too many non-clinical staff working for the NHS and the need to make cutbacks. A recent report by the department of health has suggested that one way of addressing this would be for patients to book appointments with their GPs via remote call centres, rather than through receptionists at their local surgeries. For those of you who have GP surgeries with fierce fire-breathing receptionists and phone lines that are constantly engaged, this may seem like an appealing prospect, but to me this appears to be yet another ill-thought-out attack on the fundamentals of primary care and it also clearly demonstrates a massive under-appreciation of the true value of the much-maligned GP receptionist.

At my surgery our head receptionist Sue is worth her weight in gold, and I for one would fight tooth and nail not to lose her. She has had minimal formal training and gets paid less than £9 per hour, but her value to the doctors, nurses, patients and general smooth running of the practice is immeasurable. Sue has been working at our surgery forever and she seems to have a personal relationship with almost every one of our patients. Sue knows that Mrs Walsh never makes a fuss, so if she requests a home visit she really needs one. She also knows not to book in Mr Jacobs, who is a heroin addict, with the locum doctor on a Friday afternoon, as he will try and pull a fast one and get extra diazepam for the weekend. She knows that Mrs Michaels needs to be booked in to a downstairs room as she can't manage the stairs and that when Mr Chambers books in for a blood test, he needs a double appointment and a cup of sweet tea ready as he is prone to fainting dramatically at the mere sight of a needle. She has an amazing way of placating a full waiting room of fuming patients when I'm running an hour late and she always gives me an urgent call if someone looks really poorly and needs to be squeezed into an already full surgery. Admittedly, she can also occasionally fulfil the stereotype of the fierce dragon receptionist barring the path to seeing the doctor, but from our point of view, she is our only line of defence against a constant barrage of demands that without her careful triaging would mean that we would never get to go home.

Another factor from this report appears to be the misunderstanding of how primary care is managed. GP surgeries are privately-run businesses working within the NHS. We make our own decisions about how we organise appointment systems and reception areas. Paying idle receptionists to sit around reading magazines and drinking tea really isn't in our interests. On the rare occasions that the front desk and phones are quiet, our receptionists are sorting the post, processing repeat prescription requests or calling patients in for blood tests and blood pressure checks. There are some really quite entrepreneurial penny-pinching GPs out there and if there was a way of outsourcing booking appointments without compromising patient care, it would have been done by now. At our surgery we have introduced an on-line booking system to try and take some pressure off the phone lines and make life easier for our patients. This is great for the 30-year-old who wants to book an appointment next Thursday to discuss his possible lactose intolerance, but when 93-year-old Ethel phones from the floor of her living room, unable to get up after yet another fall, she needs to speak to Sue, rather than a call centre operator hundreds of miles away.

So if we are going to reduce the amount that we spend on non-clinical staff in the NHS how are we going to do it? Well, in my surgery we have 2 managers and 2 doctors. This is clearly a ridiculous ratio. One of our managers is the practice manager. She organises the staff, deals with complaints, pays the bills and makes sure that we don't run out of toilet roll. She manages the day-to-day running of the business so that we doctors can get on with seeing patients and it would be really hard to function without her. The other manager is basically our 'targets manager'. She works nearly full time simply making sure that we reach all our targets set from above so we make enough points – and therefore money – to keep the practice running. I've droned on about these targets before so will try not to repeat myself too much. Suffice to say that they seem to change and become more numerous every year and an increasing number of hoops need to be jumped through in order for them to be met. Many targets seem to have very little direct impact on patient care, but we are paying a near full-time member of staff to make sure all of this data is correctly recorded and audited.

So if the government decides that General Practice is too expensive and they are going to give practices like mine a little less money each year, please take away some of the hoops we have to jump through and reduce the number of targets we have to reach. We can afford to lose backroom personnel like 'targets managers' but we can't afford to lose receptionists like Sue. She's a front line member of staff and a vital member of our team. She is much much more than a faceless voice on a phone tapping names into appointment slots and no, she can't be replaced by a stranger in a call centre hundreds, or even thousands of miles away.

Fit to work?

Ken is my first patient of the morning and he is not a happy bunny. The nurse at the 'fit to work assessment' has decided that he is in fact fit to work and cancelled his benefits payments. Ken is one of the 78 per cent of people that are signed off sick but are apparently entirely capable of an honest day's work. This would suggest that I and my GP colleagues' assessments of our patients' capability to work is only correct 22 per cent of the time. My doctor ego can just about cope with this sort of poor strike rate, but I'm not sure it will ever recover from having my apparent poor assessment being corrected by a nurse! The nurse who filled in a form and ruled Ken fit to work has, in a single appointment, overridden the years of sick notes that I have been dishing out.

Ken is 54 years old and is the sort of person that the government desperately wants to get back into work. He had worked as a scaffolder since leaving school at 16, but after 38 years of hard graft his shoulder gave in and he came to see me. Initially I signed him off for a week so he could rest it. That turned into a few more weeks as I organised an X-ray and physiotherapy. By the time he had seen the orthopaedic surgeon he had been off for a few months and his company had let him go. In reality, it didn't really need a specialist to tell Ken that after 38 years of back-breaking manual labour, he wasn't really up to lugging great big tubes of metal around on his shoulders any more.

We did talk about other things Ken might do but he told me that he 'wasn't the sort of bloke to work in an office'. He had worked as a scaffolder and on building sites all his life and stubborn bugger that he was, he wasn't going to consider anything else. £65.45 per week isn't a lot of money but as long as Ken had his housing benefit paid and had a small amount of pocket money for beers and cigs he was prepared to take what he called early retirement. 'There are no jobs out there for people like me' he would say and he is probably right. Ken is physically capable of working in an office, but then if 30-year-old law graduates can't get low paid admin work in an office, Ken had no chance. Judge me if you wish, but I carried on signing Ken off and he hasn't worked for the last three years.

The general consensus appears to be that as a GP I am best placed to make an informed and objective decision about my patients' capability to work. The truth is that I can't make an objective decision because I have a relationship with my patients. I have known Ken and his family for years. I have seen him cry when his mum died and shared the joy of meeting his first granddaughter. We've discussed his erectile dysfunction at great (and not so great) length and on more than one occasion I've stuck my finger up his bum. I am not a faceless nurse working for the department of work and pensions, I am his family doctor and he expects me to be on his side.

This may sound like I'm trying to defend a generation of GPs who have consistently colluded with their patients to cheat the taxpayer, but the truth is that I am the patient's advocate and without wishing to spout too much psycho-babble, I probably went into medicine partly because I wanted to be liked. It takes about ten years to train to be a GP and costs the taxpayer lots of money. There must be better ways to spend my working day than having stand-up rows with my patients over sick notes. GPs like me who work in deprived areas spend a huge amount of their time filling in sick notes and completing incapacity benefit forms. It is dull and takes appointment time away from people who need to see a doctor because they have something wrong with their health.

I do actually try and persuade many of my patients that working might be good for both their physical and mental health, but if a person has decided that they don't want to work it is very difficult for me to persuade them otherwise. If a patient tells me truthfully or otherwise that the severity of his back pain is 11 on a scale of 1–10, or that his depression is so severe that during every waking minute he considers throwing himself off a bridge, it is very hard for me to try and persuade him that he is in fact fully capable of spending an eight-hour shift on the till at Morrisons.

I am still quite young and not particularly worldly, but in my limited experience of life it strikes me that carrots work better than sticks. The cost of processing Ken's sick notes, incapacity forms, fitness to work assessments and then his appeals against the fitness to work decisions are massive. Ultimately if after this entire costly process Ken was eventually forced on to Job Seekers Allowance, the result would be that he would be getting his £65.45 from a different department but it would still be extremely unlikely that he would end up with a job. If it was up to me, rather than trying to beat Ken into submission, I would try and offer a few carrots instead. Perhaps offer him free training to go on a fork-lift driver course. Maybe offer him an extra £20 per week on top of his benefits to do six hours a week helping out at a local community centre. Getting some self-esteem back and re-entering the world of work at some level would surely push Ken closer to leaving

the benefits system than simply spending a lot of time, money
and effort switching him from one handout to another and
labelling him as a 'benefits cheat'.

Royal Wedding

I was trying to look after Bernie's blood pressure and cholesterol and was explaining that my overall aim was to keep him alive and healthy for as long as possible. 'Yes please,' Bernie replied. 'What I really want is to stay alive long enough for the royal wedding in April.'

I was really touched by this. I'm not a great royalist myself, but it seemed sweet that this nice old boy wanted to stay alive long enough to watch our future heir marry. 'I'm looking forward to the big day and settling down with a pot of Vaseline and some tissues,' Bernie told me. I must have looked slightly puzzled, so in order to clarify Bernie made his intentions crystal clear by demonstrating the universal hand symbol for masturbation.

In an awkward fluster I quickly changed the subject, but now wish I hadn't. There are so many questions that I now want the answer to. Was it just this specific royal wedding that excited him or had he also indulged for Di, Fergie and Camilla? Was it the prospect of Kate in her dress that was stirring him or was it the whole pomp and ceremony that floated his boat? For the sake of Wills, Kate and us all, I hoped that he was in fact planning to enjoy the wedding from the privacy of his own lounge and hadn't in fact been invited to Westminster Abbey as some sort of old chum of Prince Philip.

As the royal wedding came and went and we all watched endless re-runs on TV, I thought about Bernie and felt pleased that I had at least helped keep him alive long enough to enjoy his and their big day. In this age of the internet with millions of sexual images available instantly at the click of a mouse, it seemed sweet that this old boy was waiting for a royal wedding to get his libido racing. Perhaps knocking one out over a royal wedding is the ultimate demonstration of patriotism and national pride. In fact if you managed to get through watching the whole ceremony without even a vague stirring down below, perhaps you don't love your country quite as much as you thought you did.

Abortion

An argument between a mother and her 16-year-old daughter was being played out in front of me during a busy Monday morning surgery. It was like any other parent–adolescent quarrel, except for the significant issue at stake. They were arguing over whether 16- year-old Lauren should have an abortion or not.

'Tell her, Dr Daniels. Tell her she has to get rid of it. There ain't no room for a little one in our flat. I was only 16 when I 'ad Lauren so I know how hard it is. Tell her she's too young to 'ave a baby.'

I gently explained to Lauren and her mum that as her GP I would support her in whatever decision she made but that I couldn't promote one choice or the other. This is of course the professional approach to take but having recently become a parent myself, decisions about abortions can't help but be emotive on many levels. Firstly, I now understand how arduous it is to be a parent and looking at Lauren, I couldn't help but wonder how well this girl – who is in many ways still a child herself – would manage. Also, there is the matter of how I would react if my own daughter came to me aged 16 telling me she was pregnant. It was clearly heart-breaking for Lauren's mum to watch her daughter following in her own footsteps when I'm sure she had very different hopes and aspirations for her. Finally, having recently wondered in amazement at the detail seen during the antenatal scans during my wife's pregnancy, I can't ignore the reality that within Lauren there lies some form of separate entity which has its own heart-beat and with every passing day becomes that little bit closer to resembling a baby.

I can't offer an exact time as to when I believe a bunch of cells becomes a life, but I do find it more of a struggle referring late abortions in comparison to early ones. I recently saw a young woman who was pregnant but was not sure about the dates of her last period. She told me that if she was just 10 weeks pregnant she wanted an abortion but if she was 14 weeks pregnant she would allow the pregnancy to continue. I naïvely assumed that this deci-sion was being made for ethical reasons and tried in vain to engage her in a chat about embryology and the important stages of fetal development. She politely interrupted me to explain that if the embryo was 14 weeks old it was her fiancé's and she wanted to keep it and if it was 10 weeks old it was the outcome of a drunken holiday encounter that she wanted to forget. I quickly closed my embryology text book and ordered an ultrasound scan to date the pregnancy.

Going back to Lauren, I suggested that we make a list of the pros and cons of having a baby. To get things going in the cons list I ask about her plans for the future. I asked about college or a career or travelling. I thought back to all the things that I had wanted to do with my life aged 16. Lauren shrugged and admitted that she didn't really want to do anything. She wanted to be a mum and was determined to keep the baby – and that is exactly what she did.

The UK has the highest teenage pregnancy rate in Europe and the young girls in my practice seem to be doing their very best to help keep us right up there in pole position. For every pregnant teenager I see, it feels like a personal failure because our job as a

GP practice is to provide adequate contraception. In Lauren's case I don't think there were issues with lack of available contraception. I also don't think there was a lack of sex education at school or too much sex on TV and in the media. The sad fact is that Lauren, like many teenage girls growing up on our local estate, didn't really seem to have any aspirations to do anything more with her life other than have babies. There are no female role models around her who have done anything other than have children young and bring them up as single parents. Many of them, including Lauren's mum, have coped amazingly well and my hat goes off to them. I really hope Lauren does equally well and although I really don't want to in any way belittle the importance of being a mother, I can't help but think that the real failure was Lauren's lack of ambition to do anything else.

Taking responsibility

How much should we all as patients take responsibility over our own health care and how much should remain the responsibility of the doctor? There was a case recently where a woman presented to her GP with a breast lump. The doctor made an urgent referral to the hospital to check for breast cancer. Unfortunately the letter had the patient's house number as 16 when it should have been 1b and the letter for the breast clinic appointment went to the wrong address resulting in the appointment not being kept. Two years later the woman sadly died of breast cancer and her son successfully sued the GP for a large sum of money. The judge deemed the doctor to have been at fault for failing to 'ensure that she had attended the appointment'. This sort of decision really puts us back to the time when the doctor–patient relationship was paternalistic rather than the partnership that we are supposedly currently striving for. Surely as individuals we need to take a bit more responsibility for our own health? Without doubt, the surgery cocked up by having the wrong address on record and the doctor would have been wise to check the address with his patient when she was there, but as a few weeks turned into a few months, surely she must have realised something had gone astray. Perhaps there was a degree of denial on the patient's part? With on average of two thousand patients designated to each GP and up to forty appointments per day, a GP is hard pushed to keep track of every patient once they have left the consulting room.

Much as I sympathise with the GP mentioned above, I would like to think it wouldn't happen to me. Not because I am beyond not checking an address properly or missing out a digit on a telephone number, but because when I refer a woman with a breast lump I give them enough information to know that if they didn't hear anything within two weeks that something has gone wrong and they need to chase it up. I don't know how much or how little was discussed with the patient by the GP mentioned above, but in a doctor–patient partnership the idea is that the patient is given enough information and knowledge to be empowered and ideally share responsibility for their ongoing treatment. As a doctor this can be hard, as it is difficult to tell someone that you are referring them because you suspect they may have cancer. The alternative though is keeping the truth from them and letting them leave with enough false reassurance to think that it is ok to ignore a malignant breast lump, possibly with disastrous consequences.

France vs UK

Monique is a lovely French girl in her mid-twenties. We had always got on but unfortunately that was about to change. Monique had been struggling with a bad back for five days after trying to help her flat mate carry a washing machine up two flights of stairs. She had phoned her GP in France who had told her that she needed an MRI scan. This was the start of our regrettable falling out. I examined Monique and there was no denying that she had a stiff and sore back. There certainly wasn't any sign of a 'slipped disc' or a problem with the spine and I asked why it was she wanted an MRI scan. 'To find out what is wrong with my back,' she replied indignantly. 'But we know what is wrong with your back,' I replied. 'The muscles are a bit inflamed and you need to do some gentle stretching exercises and take some ibuprofen until it settles down.' 'But I need the scan to tell me exactly what is wrong so that my homeopath can treat my back naturally.'

I found it odd that this intelligent, educated woman thought that the 'natural' way to treat her back was to have an expensive unnecessary scan, followed by some expensive unnecessary placebos. As far as I was concerned it was actually me that was promoting the true 'natural' treatment, by encouraging her to accept that an inflamed lower back is a 'natural' response to carrying a washing machine up two flights of stairs. I was advocating that a few exercises and allowing 'natural' healing to take its course was probably the best approach to take. We could always review things if her symptoms weren't settling.

Monique wasn't happy, and she angrily explained to me that in France she would get an MRI scan and her homeopathic treatment directly from her GP. She then went on to tell me with no holds barred how far superior France was in comparison to England in almost all ways before storming out. I actually rather like France and wouldn't dispute French superiority on many levels, but despite Monique's displeasure, I don't believe that this was a case of a substandard NHS failing in comparison to a better quality French public health care system.

France spends considerably more on health care than we do here in the UK. I have never been a patient or a doctor in France so I can't really make any educated comments on the French health service overall, but the case of Monique does make me realise the value of sensible GPs keeping unnecessary investigations and treatments to a minimum, even if it does mean that some of our patients feel they are being short changed. MRI scans are great for many things and I wish I had more access to them, but if every young healthy adult with a few days of back pain got an MRI scan and homeopathic remedies on the NHS, our economy would fall into even more dire straits than it is already.

The NHS is brill

One of my patients called our much-maligned out of hours GP service last Sunday morning. Andy is a normally fit and healthy 20-year-old student and it was the morning after a big Saturday night out on the town. His housemates called the GP service as they were worried that he looked a bit off colour and was complaining of a headache. I often work that Sunday morning shift and as you arrive the list of calls that needs to be sorted form a chaotic and lengthy queue on the computer screen. With just one or two GPs covering an entire town, it is key to try and work out what is urgent and what can wait. For the GP last Sunday morning, added to his long list of calls about lost prescriptions, coughs and colds, sore ankles and urine infections, was a student with a headache after a big night out drinking. It would be easy to quickly dismiss this one as a hangover, but fortunately for Andy, the doctor suspected that something wasn't right. He left his ever-growing list of calls and visited Andy at home. He was greeted by a pale but coherent 20-year-old nursing a headache on his sofa. Again, this doctor's experience and sixth sense led him to suspect that Andy was suffering from something more than just a hang-over and gave him a jab of penicillin before calling an ambulance and sending him straight into hospital. On arriving, Andy took a turn for the worse but the expert staff in A&E and then ITU were on hand and he made a full recovery. Andy had meningococcal septicaemia and was probably just an hour or two from death, had he not received rapid and expert treatment.

If that GP hadn't visited him at home last Sunday Andy would have almost certainly died. It may well have made the national press and would have been used as another example of NHS failings and used to support claims of an overall decline in the standards of medical care in this country. I don't live in a bubble and I would be first to admit that the NHS can be a bit shit sometimes, as can some of the people who work within it. We need to look at our failings and improve, but thankfully when it was really needed last Sunday, the NHS and her staff came good. I would like to say a thank you to all those people who worked that Sunday morning to save Andy's life. Yes, they were just doing their jobs, and they were being paid out of all of our taxes, but they still made a huge difference to one young man and gave him a future that could so easily have been lost. The NHS is still amazing. I just hope that we don't lose it.

My patients are brill

Vincent was new to the practice so I was obliged to bring him in for a 'new patient check'. He was an African guy in his early thirties and was exceptionally polite, with an infectious broad smile. 'Any medical problems then, Vincent?' 'No, Doctor, I'm very healthy,' he beamed proudly. Vincent was good company, but his apparent first-rate healthiness was making my role as his new doctor feel superfluous. 'Oh, but there is just one thing you should probably know about, Doctor,' and with that, Vincent lifted up his shirt to reveal multiple criss-crossing scars that covered his entire abdomen.

'I thought you hadn't had any medical problems. What on earth happened there?'

'Unfortunately it was not an illness that caused these scars, Dr Daniels. I'm from Rwanda, do you know much about our troubled history?'

'Wasn't there some sort of civil war between the Hutus and the Tutsis?' I mumble.

'Well yes, Doctor, but actually it was a bit more complicated than that.'

Vincent goes on to tell me his remarkable story and that of his homeland. As the teenage son of a police chief he was a target

373

for militias on both sides, and he spent months escaping attacks by either fleeing or hiding and was left helpless as other members of his immediate family were murdered. He was finally found by one of the gangs and sustained a machete attack so vicious that his abdomen was left sliced open, leaving his intestines spilling out of him. He was left for dead, but was saved by the compassion and bravery of two of his neighbours. He tells me that they used electrical tape to try and hold his abdomen together whilst they risked their own lives driving him to the Red Cross. Other than three of his cousins, no other member of his family survived the atrocities. Vincent somehow managed to recover both physically and emotionally and has rebuilt his life. After studying and working in Belgium for some years he gained EU citizenship and decided to move to the UK and is training to be a maths teacher.

That morning a man had wanted me to sign him off sick with post-traumatic stress disorder because of someone writing mean things about him on Facebook. Vincent had experienced a level of fear and loss that I couldn't even begin to imagine, yet he was bravely making the most of his life and moving on as best he could.

By the time Vincent had finished his story I felt humbled, and as he got up to leave I asked him if there was anything I could help him with.

'Just one thing I need some help with, Dr Daniels, I'm looking for a wife. Do you know any nice single ladies?' He gave me a wink and flashed me that broad smile one last time.

When sometimes feeling downtrodden by blood pressure targets, diabetes pathways and commissioning audits, my patients never fail to offer a gentle reminder that actually everything else is a minor distraction from the true joy of the job, which is the people who sit before me and allow me to share their stories. It would be a grim job without you. Thank you!

Acknowledgements

A big thank you to my parents, Sarah and my brother for all their advice and help. Thanks to Dr Nick Edwards, who helped persuade me to write this book. Feel free to read his book *In Stitches*. It is like mine but not as good. Finally, a massive thank you to my wonderful wife, who has supported me through the writing of this book and, more importantly, through the highs and lows of life. I love you deeply.

Confessions of a GP is part of the 'Confessions' series.
Also including *Confessions of a Male Nurse*
by Michael Alexander.

'A fantastic read. Everything I had always suspected
about nurses and so much more!'
DR BENJAMIN DANIELS, author of bestselling
CONFESSIONS OF A GP

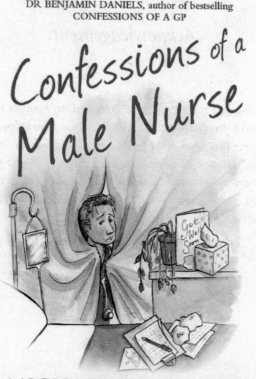

Confessions of a
Male Nurse

MICHAEL ALEXANDER

And, coming soon:
Confessions of a New York Taxi Driver
Confessions of a Police Constable